Plants
that
Heal

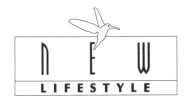

Plants
that
Heal

George D. Pamplona-Roger, M.D.

Author of the 'Encyclopedia of Medicinal Plants' and the 'Encyclopedia of Foods and Their Healing Power'
published in English, French, German, Portuguese, Italian, and Spanish

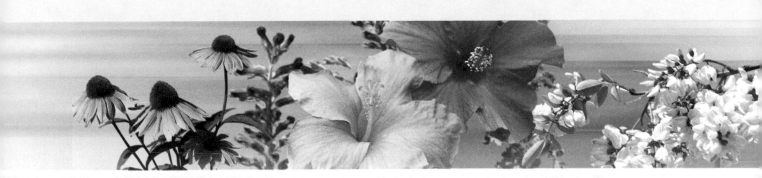

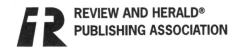

REVIEW AND HERALD®
PUBLISHING ASSOCIATION

editorial safeliz

Copyright © 2004 by **REVIEW AND HERALD PUBLISHING ASSOCIATION**
55 W. Oak Ridge Drive
Hagerstown, Maryland 21740
Phone: (301) 393 3000
e-mail: info@rpha.org – www.reviewandherald.org

ISBN 0-8280-1863-4

PRINTED IN THE UNITED STATES OF AMERICA

Editorial and Design by the editorial team of Safeliz S.L.
All drawings, images and pictures are owned by Editorial Safeliz S.L.

This magabook is an excerpt of the ENCYCLOPEDIA OF MEDICINAL PLANTS,
ISBN 84-7208-157-5, published in two volumes.
Copyright © 1995 by Editorial Safeliz S.L.
Pradillo, 6 – Polígono Industrial La Mina
28770 Colmenar Viejo, Madrid, Spain
Phone [+34] 918 459 877 – Fax [+34] 918 459 865
e-mail: admin@safeliz.com – www.safeliz.com

Notice to Readers: This magabook is designed to give information on the medicinal value of certain plants. Although the recommendations and information given are appropriate in most cases, they are of a general nature and cannot take into account the specific circumstances of individual situations. Any plant substance, used externally or internally, can cause allergic reactions in some persons. The information given in this book is not intended to take the place of professional medical care either in diagnosing or treating medical conditions. Do not attempt self-diagnosis or self-treatment for serious or long-term problems without consulting a qualified medical professional. Always seek a physician's advice before undertaking any self-treatment or if symptoms persist. Neither the publisher nor the author can assume responsibility for problems arising from the mistaken identity of any plant or from the inappropriate use made of it by readers. Advice is given in page 36 on the safe use of medical herbs.

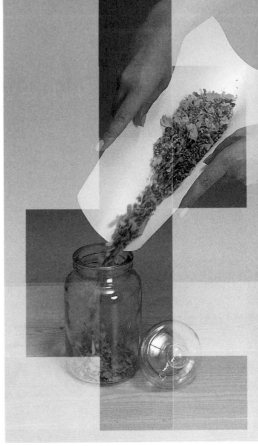

Table of Contents

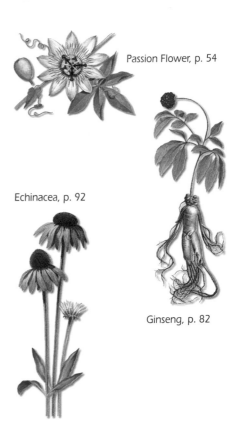

Passion Flower, p. 54

Echinacea, p. 92

Ginseng, p. 82

Meaning of the Icons of Botanical Parts
Used in This Work

In this magabook there are a number of icons, symbols,
and tables which describe plants, body organs, and ailments.
We describe these icons on the following pages so the reader can be familiar
with them and interpret their meaning more easily.

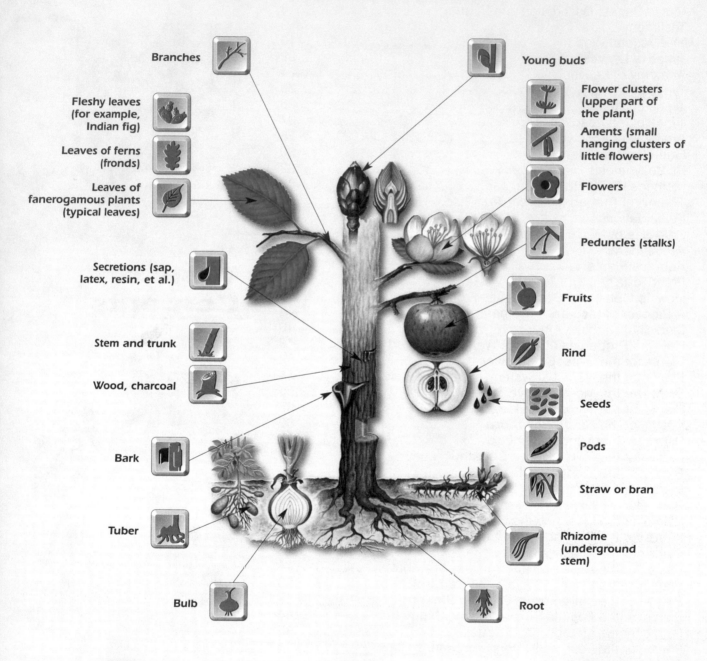

Branches

Young buds

Flower clusters (upper part of the plant)

Aments (small hanging clusters of little flowers)

Fleshy leaves (for example, Indian fig)

Leaves of ferns (fronds)

Leaves of fanerogamous plants (typical leaves)

Flowers

Peduncles (stalks)

Secretions (sap, latex, resin, et al.)

Fruits

Stem and trunk

Rind

Wood, charcoal

Seeds

Pods

Bark

Straw or bran

Tuber

Rhizome (underground stem)

Bulb

Root

Thallus (vegetative part of algae and moss)

The whole plant

The whole plant except the root

Meaning of the Icons of Anatomical Parts
Used in This Work

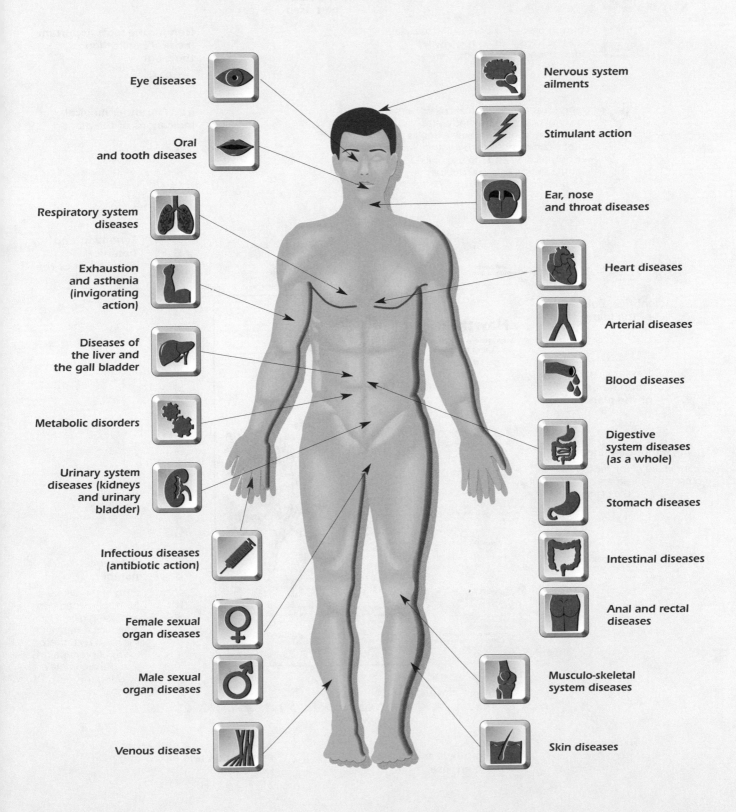

Eye diseases

Oral and tooth diseases

Respiratory system diseases

Exhaustion and asthenia (invigorating action)

Diseases of the liver and the gall bladder

Metabolic disorders

Urinary system diseases (kidneys and urinary bladder)

Infectious diseases (antibiotic action)

Female sexual organ diseases

Male sexual organ diseases

Venous diseases

Nervous system ailments

Stimulant action

Ear, nose and throat diseases

Heart diseases

Arterial diseases

Blood diseases

Digestive system diseases (as a whole)

Stomach diseases

Intestinal diseases

Anal and rectal diseases

Musculo-skeletal system diseases

Skin diseases

Plant Pages: Description and Format

Icon of plant use:

Free use: the plant has no side effects or contraindications.

Caution use: it is a potentially toxic plant. It can be used with no risk, always remembering the caution given.

Dangerous use: it is a toxic plant, with a powerful action on the body, also causing undesirable effects. In some cases, its use is not recommended, and in other cases, we only recommend the use of its pharmaceutical extracts, carefully dosed and under medical supervision.

Icon of botanical part used (see p. 6)

Chapter title

Icon for the most important medical application of the plant (see p. 7)

Icons for other medical indications of the plant (see p. 7)

Synonyms and botanical description of the plant

Scientific name of the plant

Common name of the plant

Minor heading Summary of the most outstanding features of the plant

Main text

Illustration of the plant

Reference number: Each of the different forms of preparation and use is given a reference number. In the main text, these forms of preparation and use are implied by using this number.

Warning box (if any) for the plant use

Preparation and use box

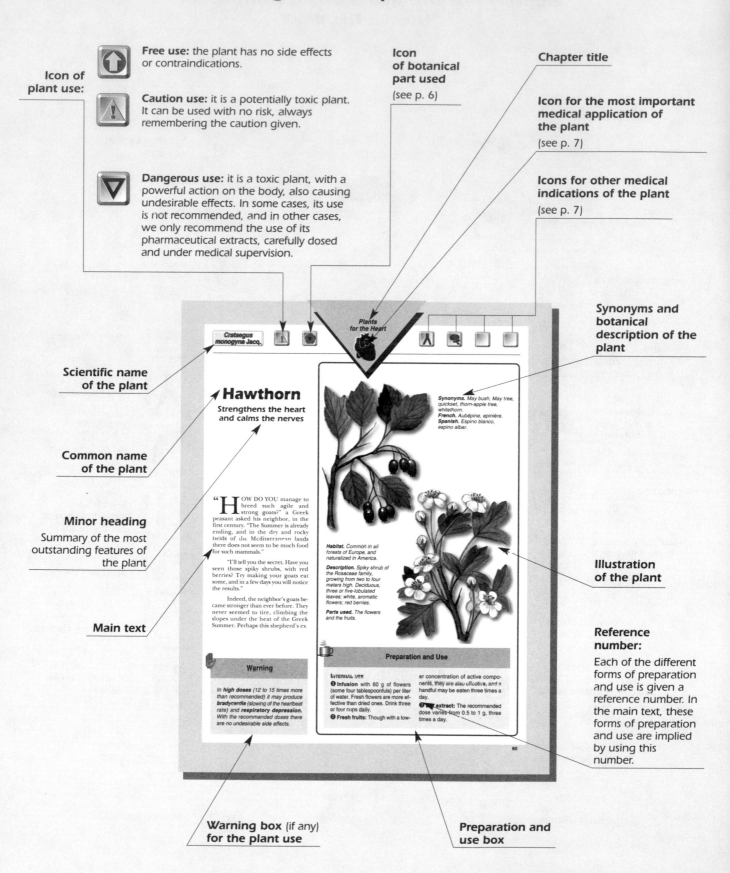

Crataegus monogyna Jacq.

Plants for the Heart

Hawthorn
Strengthens the heart and calms the nerves

"HOW DO YOU manage to breed such agile and strong goats?" a Greek peasant asked his neighbor, in the first century. "The Summer is already ending, and in the dry and rocky fields of the Mediterranean lands there does not seem to be much food for such mammals."

"I'll tell you the secret. Have you seen those spiky shrubs, with red berries? Try making your goats eat some, and in a few days you will notice the results."

Indeed, the neighbor's goats became stronger than ever before. They never seemed to tire, climbing the slopes under the heat of the Greek Summer. Perhaps this shepherd's ex

Synonyms. May bush, May tree, quickset, thorn-apple tree, whitethorn.
French. Aubépine, epinière.
Spanish. Espino blanco, espino albar.

Habitat. Common in all forests of Europe, and naturalized in America.

Description. Spiky shrub of the Rosaceae family, growing from two to four meters high. Deciduous, three or five-lobulated leaves; white, aromatic flowers; red berries.

Parts used. The flowers and the fruits.

Warning

In **high doses** (12 to 15 times more than recommended) it may produce **bradycardia** (slowing of the heartbeat rate) and **respiratory depression**. With the recommended doses there are no undesirable side effects.

Preparation and Use

INTERNAL USE
❶ **Infusion** with 60 g of flowers (some four tablespoonfuls) per liter of water. Fresh flowers are more effective than dried ones. Drink three or four cups daily.
❷ **Fresh fruits:** Though with a low-er concentration of active components, they are also effective, and a handful may be eaten three times a day.

❸ **Dry extract:** The recommended dose varies from 0.5 to 1 g, three times a day.

60

*T*hroughout the ages, plants have been used by humans as a source of food, cosmetics and medicines, and have provided raw materials for the construction of shelters and the manufacture of clothing. The significance of tropical forests in the maintenance of the earth's ecological balance is only now being fully appreciated and understood. There is an urgent need to conserve and use these resources in an environmentally sustainable and economically beneficial manner.

Plants have served as the basis of sophisticated traditional medicine systems for thousands of years in countries such as China and India. These plant-based systems continue to play an essential role in health care. It has been estimated by the World Health Organization that about 80% of the world's inhabitants rely mainly on traditional medicines for their primary health care.

Plant products also play an important role in the health care systems of the remaining 20 percent of the population who mainly reside in developed countries. Analysis of data on prescriptions dispensed from community pharmacies in the United States from 1959 to 1980 indicates that about 25 percent contained plant extracts or active components derived from higher plants. At least 119 chemical substances, derived from 90 plant species, can be considered as important drugs currently in use in one or more countries.

The United States National Cancer Institute (NCI) was established in 1937, its mission being "to provide for, foster, and aid in coordinating research related to cancer." The NCI has screened well over 100,000 plant extracts for anticancer activity and over 30,000 for anti-AIDS activity.

The development of clinically effective anticancer agents such as taxol, and the discovery of potential anti-AIDS agents such as michellamine B, demonstrate the value of plants as sources of potential new drugs, and highlight the importance of conserving these valuable resources.

TESTIMONY

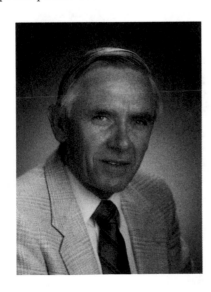

Dr. Gordon M. Cragg
Natural Products Branch,
U. S. National Cancer
Institute

THE VEGETAL WORLD

"What a surprise! This piece of cork is formed by thousands of tiny cells, joined together. It resembles a honeycomb!" said Robert Hooke, a famous seventeenth century English physicist, astonished by what he saw through his microscope.

His scientific spirit surprised him at what others would not even have noticed. Hooke had just discovered that living tissues are not a uniform and continuous mass, such as stones or minerals, but a mass made of innumerable little independent units.

"Since these little cavities form cork, I will call them cells," Hooke said. "Besides, the Latin word *cellula* means little cavity."

Cells: The Units of Life

When studying other plants under the microscope, scientists noticed that not only the bark of cork oak trees was formed by cells. All living beings, vegetals and animals, are formed by one or many grouped cells.

Each cell is a life unit. It is the smallest part of a living being that has its own life, that is to say, cells are born, get fed, grow, reproduce themselves and die.

The size of cells generally varies in a range between five and 50 microns (a thousandth of millimeter), which means that in one millimeter there may be from 20 to 200 cells, depending on their size.

Some cells will only live for a few minutes, continually being renewed, while others live as long as the living being of which they are part.

Cell Constitution

Each and every cell is formed by:

- A **nucleus,** which keeps the genetic information it has inherited, and in which all its features are printed under the guise of chromosome and genes. These will be transmitted to the next generation of cells.

- **Cytoplasm,** of viscous consistency, similar to egg white, where all biochemical processes take place.

- A cytoplasmic **membrane,** which com-

The Vegetal Cell

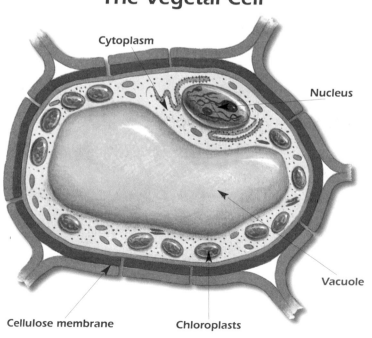

Cytoplasm

Nucleus

Vacuole

Cellulose membrane

Chloroplasts

pletely surrounds the cell and filters in a selective way all those substances which may penetrate the interior.

Features of Vegetal Cells

Vegetal cells present two basic features which cannot be found in animal cells:

1. A Cellulose Membrane

It is a thick cell wall, located outside and around the cytoplasmic membrane and is made of cellulose. It is like a porous case which isolates and protects the cell, and remains when it dies, becoming a kind of sarcophagus. Animal cells do not have any such thick cellulose membrane, therefore when they die they rot and leave no remains.

Adult cell membranes may contain other substances apart from cellulose:

- **Lignin** in wood cells.
- **Suberin** in suber, or cork cells.
- **Pectin** or **cutin,** in the cuticle which covers young stems and leaves.

Thus, what Hooke observed through the microscope—cork—were not bark cells of the cork oak tree, but their cases or cell membranes, which remain after the cell dies. Wood is also formed by the thick cellulose and lignin walls which once covered the now-already-dead stem cells.

2. Plasts

This is another peculiar feature of vegetal cells. Plasts are corpuscles located inside the cytoplasm, which contain diverse coloring substances. The most common ones are **chloroplasts,** green-colored because of their chlorophyll content.

Photosynthesis takes place inside the chloroplasts. This is an extraordinary chemical reaction where the inorganic mineral substances of air and soil turn into starch and other organic substances, thanks to sunlight energy.

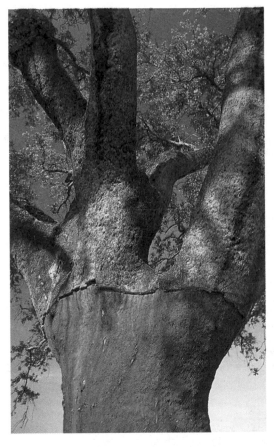

By observing cork, which comes from cork oak tree bark, through the microscope, Robert Hooke discovered in the seventeenth century that living tissues are made of tiny units called cells.

Vegetal cells differ from animal cells in that they are surrounded by a thick cellulose wall which covers them, and contain chloroplasts filled with chlorophyll. Thus, cellulose (also called vegetal fiber) and chlorophyll are the most representative substances of the vegetal world.

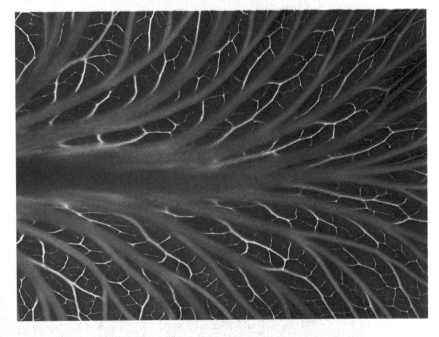

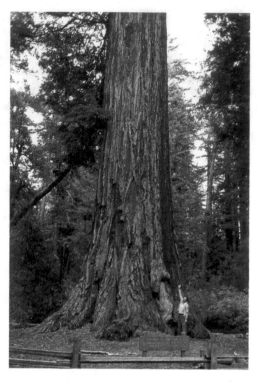

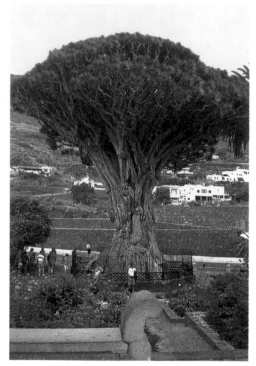

Left: **The huge sequoias of the Californian forests are regarded as being some of the tallest trees on our planet.**

Right: **The island of Tenerife, Canary Islands, houses several dragon trees such this one, trees old up to 5000 years.**

Cells are fantastic chemical laboratories. In each of them, despite their tiny size, thousands of chemical reactions take place, and their result is the synthesis of sugars (carbohydrates), lipids (fats), and proteins, which either accumulate inside the cell or flow outside it.

Alkaloids, essences and other active principles, also produced in vegetal cells, are stored inside cavities located in the cytoplasm which are called **vacuoles.** When these vacuoles break because of pressure exerted on any of the vegetable parts, the active principles they contain break free.

Diversity of the Vegetal Kingdom

"These bricks are for building the outer walls, those for covering the inner rooms, those tiles are for the kitchen floor…."

An architect gives appropriate orders so that each and every one of the hundreds and even thousands of elements that form the house goes to its appropriate place. When the building is finished, everyone will acknowledge the work of the man who designed the house and supervised the work.

However, very few people are conscious of the admirable fact that the billions of "bricks," that is to say, cells, that form a plant or any other living being are perfectly disposed each one in its place, and all of them in good working order. Who was the architect or engineer that designed this? Who directed the work? Why do epidermic cells always gather in order to cover leaves and stems? Why do hollow and elongated cells join each other to form the vessels through which sap flows?

Vegetables are living beings made of vegetal cells. Some vegetables consist of a single cell (**unicellular**), such as bacteria and certain types of fungi and algae. Others consist of many cells (**multicellular**), such as common seaweeds and mushrooms, and all superior vegetables or plants.

Size Diversity

The size of vegetables may range from a few microns, such as microorganisms, to more than 80 meters, such as the huge Californian sequoias, and to even 150 meters such as the giant Australian eucalyptus, which are regarded as being the tallest trees in the world. But there is a vegetable which still exceeds these sizes: the giant sargasso, a seaweed that may reach up to 300 meters.

Volume Diversity

As for volume, the biggest tree in the world, and probably the oldest (it is supposed to be from 4000 to 5000 years old) is the Cypress of Moctezuma, which grows in the cemetery of Santa María de Tule, in the Mexican state of Oaxaca. The spanish conquistador Hernán Cortés and his troops camped under its immense, unique crown with a diameter of 132 meters, in the year 1519.

Habitat Diversity

Some plants grow in water, such as watercresses and water lilies; others grow in desert areas, such as the agave and the aloe; some of them grow in cold climates, such as blueberries and raspberry canes; others grow in warm climates, such as the lavender and the fig tree; some in polar zones, such as moss and lichen; others in tropical areas, such as the avocado tree and the guaiac.

Diversity of the Life Span

Vegetable life widely varies. Some bacteria live only for a few minutes; Bermuda grass and other lawns may just live for a few days when there is drought. However, fir

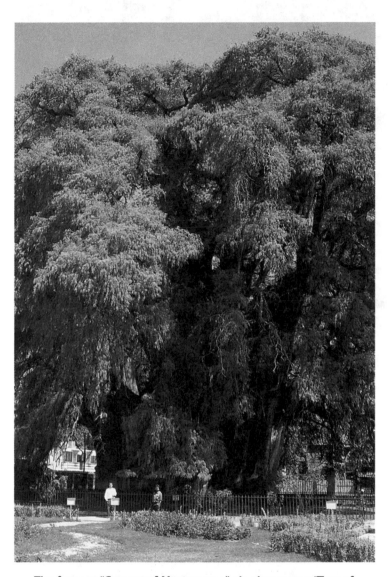

The famous "Cypress of Moctezuma," also known as "Tree of Tule," grows in the beautiful Mexican state of Oaxaca. According to the information offered to visitors, it is 41.8 meters high and its gigantic trunk reaches 14 meters in diameter. Its volume is calculated to be 816.8 cubic meters, weighing 636.1 tons, and is thus the most voluminous tree in the world (though not the tallest), and probably the heaviest and most voluminous living thing on planet Earth (the largest whales do not exceed 150 tons in weight).

Botanically it is an ahuehuete, a variety of cypress, of the family of Taxodiaceae.

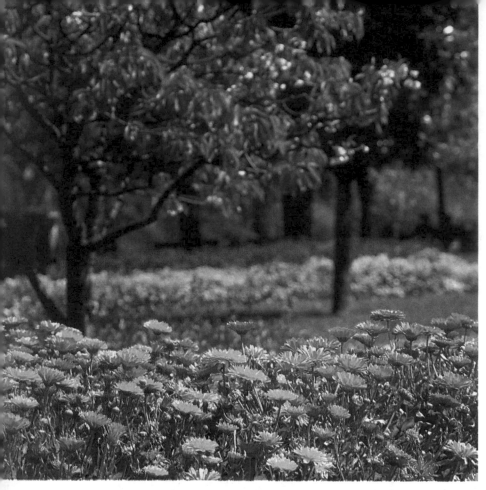

The whole earth is an immense garden, or at least that was the wish of its Creator. However, besides being ornamental, flowers and plants, many of them with medicinal properties, greatly contribute to the welfare and health of humanity.

trees live up to 800 years, and chestnut and olive trees can live for one thousand years.

In a graveyard in Yorkshire, England, there is a yew tree which is supposed to be 3000 years old. There are sequoias in California and baobabs in Africa which are over 4000 years old. These venerable trees are still alive having witnessed the rise and fall of great empires and civilizations, as well as many different human works.

However, the lifetime record is held by a dragon tree which grew in La Orotava Valley, on the island of Tenerife, Spain. This tree was uprooted in 1868 by a hurricane. In its trunk, more than 5000 rings were observed (reflecting 5000 years of age!). No other tree is known to have exceeded that age.

Structure Diversity: *From a Single Cell to Millions*

- The simplest vegetables or **schizophytes** consist of a single cell of microscopic

size. Among them, the spirulin (an alga) has outstanding medicinal properties. When we eat it, we are consuming millions of individual cells, all of them identical. It is quite logical that we are unable to distinguish any different parts in these living beings.

- **Thallophytes** are vegetables whose body or thallus usually consists of multiple different cells, yet similar to each other. These plants do not have true tissues and organs, nor roots, stems, leaves or flowers. This is demonstrated in algae, fungi and lichens. The thallus of kelp, of Iceland moss, of Irish moss, and of bladder fucus, also called wrack, are used for medicinal purposes.

- **Embryophytes** are superior vegetables, commonly known as plants. They consist of millions of cells, and seventy or eighty classes may be observed in these vegetables. Each type of cell specializes in certain functions, thus forming the diverse organs or parts of the plant: the root, the stem, the leaves, the flowers, etc.

Shape Diversity

The shape of vegetables also presents a wide range of contrasts, varying from the delicacy of a violet to the aggressiveness of a cactus; from the simplicity of thyme to the sophistication of an orchid. And what could we say about their color, about all the different green tones of their leaves, all of them similar but not exactly the same? What about the wide color range of flowers, which are made up of the entire light spectrum?

Have you ever seen an unpleasant plant? In all of the immense richness of their shapes, colors and tones, each vegetable keeps harmony, a charm and a balance of its own. Besides, many of them serve as food and heal our diseases.

Diversity of Medicinal Properties

The great richness of the vegetal world can be seen in the many medicinal substances that plants synthesize; in a range that goes from antibiotics, such as garlic and capuchin to heart-stimulants, such as cactus and foxglove, as well as sedatives such as poppy and valerian, antirheumatics such as devil's claw, energizing such as ginseng and rosemary. Their scope of properties practically meets all needs. "Prairies and hills are the best pharmacies," said Paracelsus, the renowned sixteenth century Swiss naturalist and physician.

Only One Origin

Are we conscious of the merit of our house's architect? Order cannot ever be born from chaos, even after millions of years. Pure chaos just gives birth to increasing disorder.

In order to cause and keep harmony, the direct action of a Superior Intellect is needed. When penetrating deeper into the study of the vegetal world, we cannot help but acknowledge the action of the universe's Creator, who designed the "buildings" (living entities) and distributed their "bricks" (cells) in perfect order.

Parts of the Plants

Active substances are unequally distributed among the diverse parts or organs of a plant, because of the specialization of its cells. Knowing that valerian has sedative properties is not enough: we must know which part of the plant should be used. In some cases, all parts of a plant contain the same active principles, and there is no difference in which part we use. However, of it, we may also find the following cases:

- That medicinal active ingredients are concentrated in **a single part** of a plant, for instance, only ginseng root contains invigorating substances.

- That **each part** of a plant produces **different substances,** and therefore has different properties. On orange trees, the flowers are sedative and the fruits are invigorating, while the orange tree bark has digestive and appetizer properties.

- That **some parts** of a plant produce **medicinal substances,** while **other** produce **toxic elements** instead. This is the case with the root of common comfrey, which is an excellent cicatrizant (wound healing agent) because of its content in alantoine, while its stem and leaves contain a toxic alkaloid that makes these parts quite poisonous.

The WHO (World Health Organization) considers as a "medicinal herb" any vegetable containing in one or more of its organs, any substance that can be used with therapeutical aims, or as raw material for chemical-pharmaceutical synthesis.

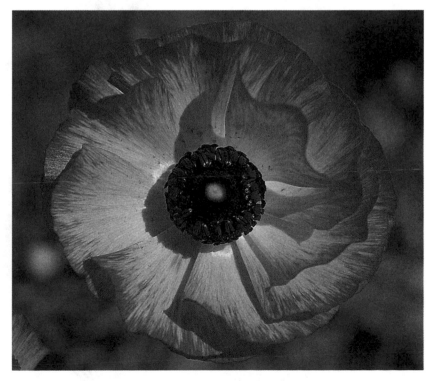

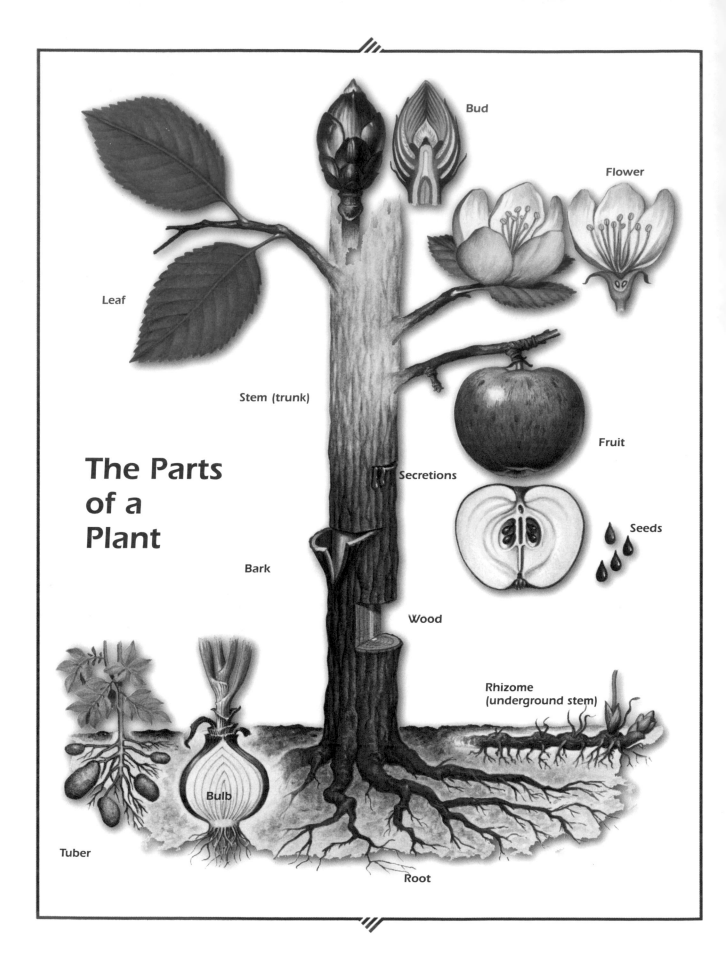

Bud

Flower

Leaf

Stem (trunk)

**The Parts
of a
Plant**

Secretions

Fruit

Bark

Seeds

Wood

Rhizome
(underground stem)

Bulb

Tuber

Root

Therefore, and according to what we have said, you should know and be able to identify each one of the parts or organs of a plant.

The Root

The root is the organ in charge of absorbing water and minerals from the soil, and pumping them up to the leaves in order to feed the whole plant. All plants usually produce starch, inuline and other sugars (also known as carbohydrates), which are stored in the roots, as in the case of chicory, artichokes, burdock, carline, dandelion, echinacea, jalap, rhatany, and yellow goatsbeard.

The root of other plants, however, also synthesize alkaloids (for example, ipecac, rauwolfia), glycosides (for example, monkshood, hound's tongue, echinacea, saxifrage) or vitamins (such as carrots).

In some cases only the root bark is useful, because the active components are more concentrated in it. This is the case of the guava tree, common barberry, boxwood, and New Jersey Tea.

The Rhizome

The rhizome is an underground stem which looks like a root, but actually grows horizontally instead of vertically. It also stores carbohydrates and nutrients as well as active components. In many cases (bistort, sweet flag, turmeric, witch grass, iris, female fern, rhubarb), the rhizome is preferred to true roots.

The Bulb

The bulb is an underground stem which consists of many overlaying layers. Sulphur essences (garlic, onion), aromatic substances (Madonna lily) or alkaloids (meadow saffron) can be found in bulbs.

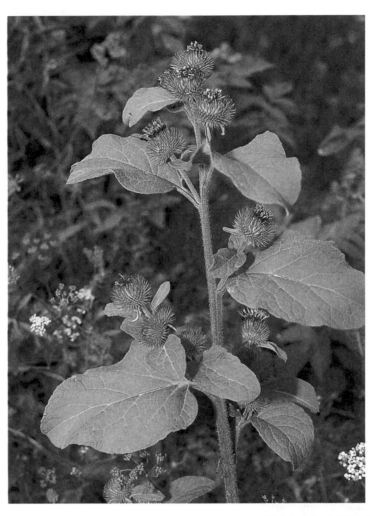

The burdock ("Arctium lappa" L.) is one of the plants whose root is richest in active components: it contains antibiotic, diuretic and hypoglycemiant (which diminish the level of sugar in the blood) substances.

The Tuber

A tuber is an underground stem which specializes in storing reserve substances, for instance, that of the early purple orchid, whose tubers produce a medicinal flour.

The Bark

The bark is a layer which covers the stem and the roots. Many active substances are stored in it (common alder, cinnamon tree, sacred bark, condurango, alder buckthorn, cinchona, oak tree, yaw tree, etc.)

17

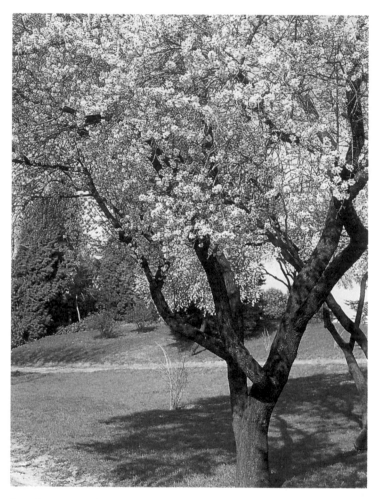

Apart from beauty and a fine scent, flowers provide diverse active components with medicinal action: essential oils, alkaloids, pigments, and glycosides.

Bud

Each bud is a would-be branch, leaf or flower. It contains essences and resins. Phytotherapy uses, for instance, buds of the silver birch, the fir tree, the black poplar and the pine tree.

Leaves

The leaves are a kind of chemical laboratory for the plant, where **photosynthesis** takes place. Photosynthesis is the whole set of chemical processes by which the plant produces complex chemical substances from inorganic substances of the air and the soil. The cells of leaves contain chlorophyll, a substance that absorbs sunlight energy, turning it into chemical energy.

The leaves **produce most of the plant's active components,** especially alkaloids, essences, glycosides and tannins. Therefore, leaves are **the most used parts of medicinal herbs.** Some of the most useful leaves in phytotherapy are those of aloe, hazelnut tree, boldo, Mexican damiana, foxglove, bearberry, witch hazel, laurel, mistletoe, chestnut tree, olive tree, grapevine and bramble.

Flowers

Flowers are the reproductive organs of plants. They contains many active components: **essential oils** (false acacia, Madonna lily, capuchin, tansy, yaw tree), **alkaloids** (poppy, sand spurry, passion flower), **pigments** (corn-flower, rose), **glycosides** (cactus, calendula, hops, orange tree, black elder), and many others.

- **Stigma.** From some flowers, as in the case of saffron or corn, only stigmas are used (stigmas are the upper parts of the female reproduction organs of flowers, called pistils).

- **Amentus.** These are pendular bunches of almost always unisexual flowers, those of hazelnut trees are an example of the most used ones.

The Stem

The stem is a kind of highway connecting the root with the other parts of the plant. In some cases it contains active components (artichokes, sugar cane, spiked alpinia, horsetail, ephedra, asparagus). Stems can be **herbaceous** (in so-called herbaceous plants) or **woody** (made of wood) as in trees and shrubs. Wood is used because of its essences (camphor tree, cypress, quassia, guaiac), besides serving as charcoal after being burnt (black poplar, common beech).

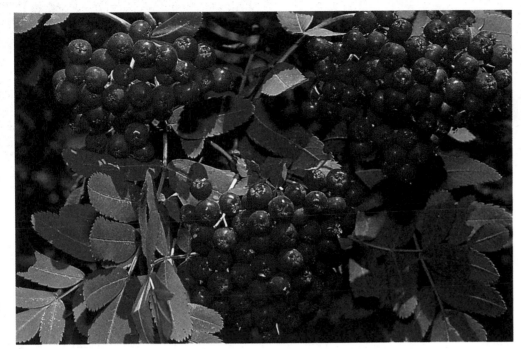

Fruits contain, generally, vitamins, mineral salts, sugars and organic acids. Some fruits, such as those of the rowan ("Sorbus aucuparia" L.) also contain pectin, a vegetal fiber with a laxative action, and tannins with astringent properties. The result of such a combination of active components is a regulating and normalizing effect for intestinal digestion.

Fruits

The fruits are those vegetal organs which grow from flowers and cover seeds.

Fleshy fruits contain abundant **organic acids,** sugars and vitamins (common barberry, bilberry, caimito, cherry, hawthorn, black elder, bramble). Others are **dry fruits,** such as those of the *Umbelliferae* family, and contain **essential oils** (anise, cumin, parsley), while some are used because of their **latex** (opium poppy).

Berries are fleshy fruits which do not have pits.

Stalks

Stalks, also called peduncles, are the parts which hold flowers, fruits, or leaves (in this case called **petioles**) from a branch or stem. Those of the cherry and Venus' hair are used in phytotherapy.

Clusters

Clusters are the upper parts of a plant in which little leaves and flowers grow together. These are used together (wormwood, heather, wild marjoram, rosemary, thyme, European golden-rod, and in general all plants of the family of *Labiatae*). When these clusters consist of flowers in their main part, they are called **flower clusters.**

The Seed

In each seed there is a future plant, as well as one or two **cotyledons** containing nourishing substances. Seeds give **sugars and lipids** (hazelnut tree, oat, cocoa, corn, chestnut), **mucilages** (fenugreek, flax, fleawort) and **oil** (opium poppy, flax, fever plant, castor bean, grapevine).

Cereal seeds are called **grains.**

Secretions

Secretions cannot be regarded as proper parts of a plant, because they consist of liquid substances, more or less viscous, produced by vegetables.

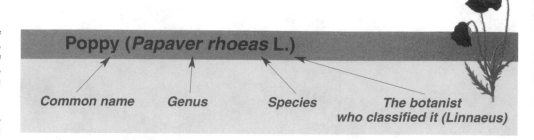

Poppy (*Papaver rhoeas* L.)

Common name   Genus   Species   The botanist who classified it (Linnaeus)

- **Latex,** milky in color and different from sap (opium poppy, celandine, fig tree, bitter lettuce, papaya).
- **Resin,** which is rich in balsamic essences (fir tree, asafetida, copal tree, guaiac, lentiscus, pine tree, etc.).
- **Sap,** which is the nutritive liquid of the plant (silver birch, agave, grapevine).

The Names of the Plants

How can the great variety of plants in the vegetal world be named in an orderly manner? And, how can they be classified? According to the color of their flowers, to the shape of their leaves, or maybe to the chemical substances they produce?

In ancient Greece, *Aristotle,* Theophrastus and Dioscorides thought about some plant classification and naming systems. Since then, other researchers and scientists have also tried to establish a universal system, however, with no success. Thus, the increasing number of used names and classifications made difficult any exchange of experiences, data and knowledge among botanists, pharmacists and physicians from different regions and countries.

In order to overcome this chaos, in 1753 the great Swedish naturalist and botanist Carolus Linnaeus, introduced a name and classification system for plants which has obtained worldwide recognition and success. It is called the **binomial system,** because it gives each species two names: the first is the **genus** name, while the second is the name of the **species.** Linnaeus had, like Adam in Eden, the privilege of giving names to all known plants. He used the Latin language, which, being a dead language, would not allow any deformation in names.

The common names of plants differ from one language to another. Even in the same linguistic region or area, plants are given different names. However, their Latin names, given by Linnaeus, remain

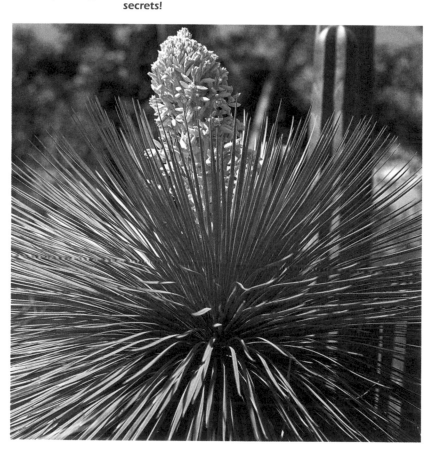

unchanged and were used worldwide. An homage to this great observer of Nature is the capitalized "L", followed by a full stop ("L.") after the scientific name of many medicinal herbs. This means that these plants were named and classified by him.

The Classification of Plants

Linnaeus classified plants according to the features of their reproduction organs. However, as botany progressed, especially by observation through microscope, the original system of Linnaeus was modified and improved till reaching its present form.

Species and its Varieties

The unit for classification is the species, which groups individuals with many similar features. Thus, the poppy (*Papaver rhoeas* L.) is, for instance, a species.

All poppies in a wheat field are alike. However, when we compare poppies growing, let us say in Spain, with those growing in Mexico, we will notice some differences. All of them are poppies, and belong to the same species, but they form different varieties.

The varieties that any species may present are a consequence of the kind of soil it grows in, of the climate and of the possible hybridizations or cross-pollinations it may have undergone. Its chemical composition is the same for all varieties, though there may be differences in the concentration of active components. Thus, for instance, the opium poppy that grows in Asia and the Middle East produces a larger amount of morphine than the European variety.

Genus

Similar species are grouped in genera. For instance, the poppy (*Papaver rhoeas* L.)

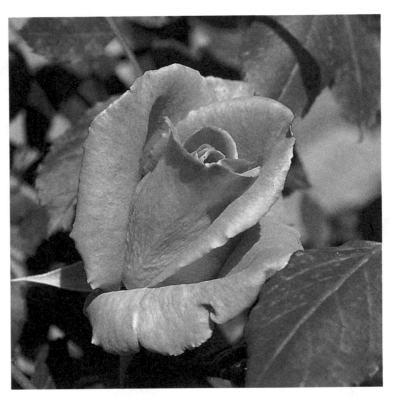

For each species there are many varieties.
For instance, the species "Rosa gallica" L. (the rose) has more than 10,000 varieties, and each of these produces roses with different features.

and the opium poppy (*Papaver somniferum* L.) belong to the same genus, *Papaver*. Both species produce similar alkaloids, though those of the opium poppy are more active.

Family

Several genera are grouped in a family. For instance, the poppy and the opium poppy, along with the greater celandine (*Chelidonium majus* L.) belong to the family of *Papaveraceae*. All of them produce a latex rich in more or less narcotic alkaloids.

Orders and Phylum

Several families are grouped in an order, the latter in classes, and classes are grouped in phylum.

Types

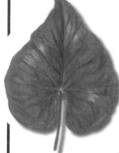

Heart-shaped
Its shape resembles a heart.

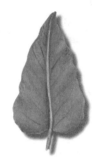

Lanceolated
Its shape resembles a spear.

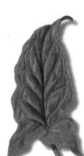

Arrow-shaped
The shape of these leaves resembles an arrow.

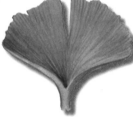

Bilobulated
This type of leaf is cut into two lobules.

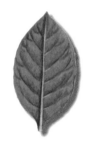

Ellipsoidal
With shape of ellipse.

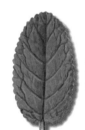

Oval
Shaped as an oval.

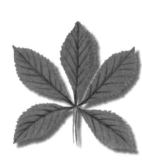

Hand-shaped
This is a compound leaf, in which the divisions are shaped like the fingers of a hand.

According to Their Nerve System

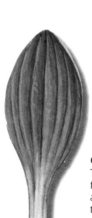

Parallelinerve
The nerves run parallel along the leaf.

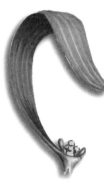

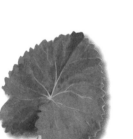

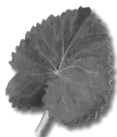

Penninerve
The nerves stem from a central axis.

Curvinerve
The nerves form a curve along the leaf.

Radial
The nerves stem as a radius from a common center.

# of Leaves

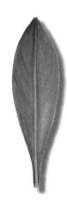

Whole
The border is
straight.

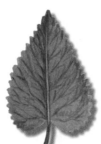

Toothed
The border
has tiny teeth.

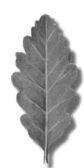

Lobulated
The border has cracks
which form lobules.

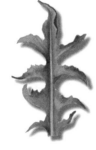

Divided
The cracks of the border
reach the central nerve.

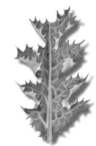

Split
The cracks of the border
almost touch the central
nerve.

According to the Position on the Stem

Petioled
These leaves join
the stem by means
of a petiole.

Alternated
These are petioled leaves which grow
one at a time along the stem.

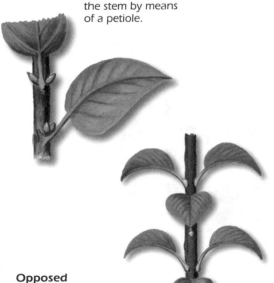

Opposed
These petioled leaves
grow in opposite pairs.

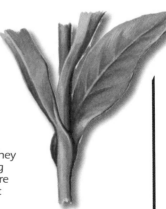

Sessile
These leaves
do not have
petiole. When they
grow embracing
the stem their are
called decurrent
leaves.

23

Anatomy of Leaves

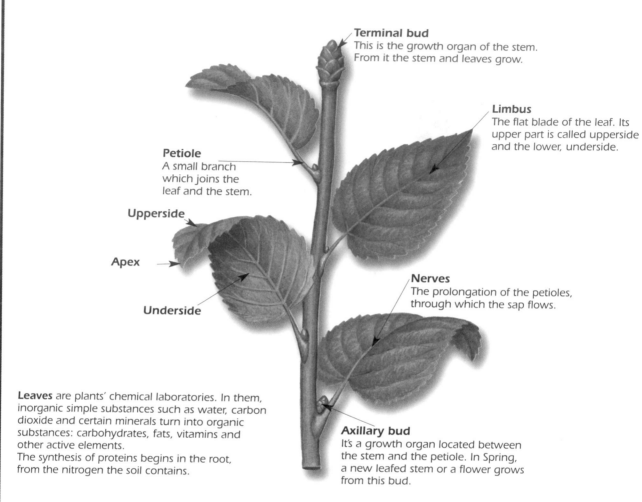

Terminal bud
This is the growth organ of the stem. From it the stem and leaves grow.

Limbus
The flat blade of the leaf. Its upper part is called upperside and the lower, underside.

Petiole
A small branch which joins the leaf and the stem.

Upperside

Apex

Underside

Nerves
The prolongation of the petioles, through which the sap flows.

Axillary bud
It's a growth organ located between the stem and the petiole. In Spring, a new leafed stem or a flower grows from this bud.

Leaves are plants' chemical laboratories. In them, inorganic simple substances such as water, carbon dioxide and certain minerals turn into organic substances: carbohydrates, fats, vitamins and other active elements.
The synthesis of proteins begins in the root, from the nitrogen the soil contains.

Microscopic Section of a Leaf

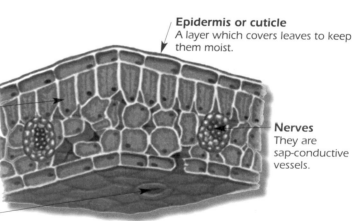

Epidermis or cuticle
A layer which covers leaves to keep them moist.

Parenchyma
Formed by cells containing abundant chlorophyll, which give leaves their green color.

Nerves
They are sap-conductive vessels.

Stomas
Little holes located in the underside of the leaf, through which carbon dioxide is absorbed and water vapor and oxygen eliminated. Stomas are surrounded by lips which act as valves, opening and closing to control the flow of gas, according to the plant's needs.

Types of Roots

Besides attaching the plant to the ground, the root absorbs nutrients and water from the earth through tiny absorbent hairs located at the tips of its branches.

Common root

Taproot

Secondary root

Absorbent hairs

Elongation region

Tuber root
It produces swellings called tubers, in which carbohydrates, proteins and other reserve nutrients are stored.

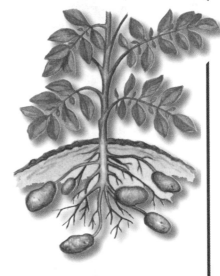

Turnip-shaped root
With a conic shape, it also stores reserve nutrients.

Fasciculated root
The secondary roots grow together at the base of the stem and are all similarly sized.

Woody root
With gross, hard ramifications.

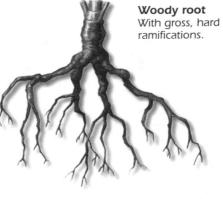

Bulb
The bulb is not actually a root, but an underground bud which consists of fleshy leaves arranged in superimposed layers.

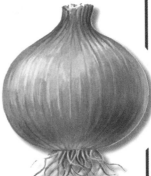

Adventitious roots
Those which grow directly from an air stem or an underground stem or rhizome.

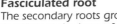

Types of Stems

The stem connects the root and the leaves,
and contains conductive vessels through which the sap flows.

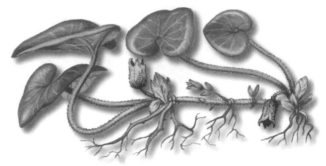

Woody stem
The cellulose which covers the cells of woody stems (trunks) is soaked with lignin.
This substance gives the cellulose the thickness of the wood.

Underground stem or rhizome
This is a stem which grows underground. Though it resembles a root, actually it is not.

Herbaceous stem
A fragile stem, because the cellulose covering its cells is not soaked with lignin. Chicory and other annual plants have this type of stem.

Succulent stem
It is sizable, spongy and without leaves. This stem stores a high amount of water, such as the cactus and other desert plants.

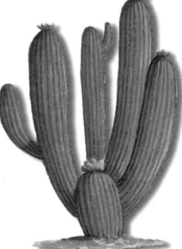

Climbing stem
This one is not consistent enough to keep itself upright, thus it grows on other plants, securing itself by means of tendrils.

Creeping stem
It grows horizontally on the ground.

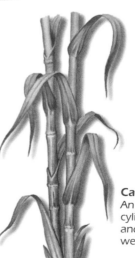

Cane
An herbaceous stem, cylinder-shaped and hollow, with well-marked nodes.

Types of Inflorescences

Inflorescences are groups of flowers which grow
from a common peduncle.

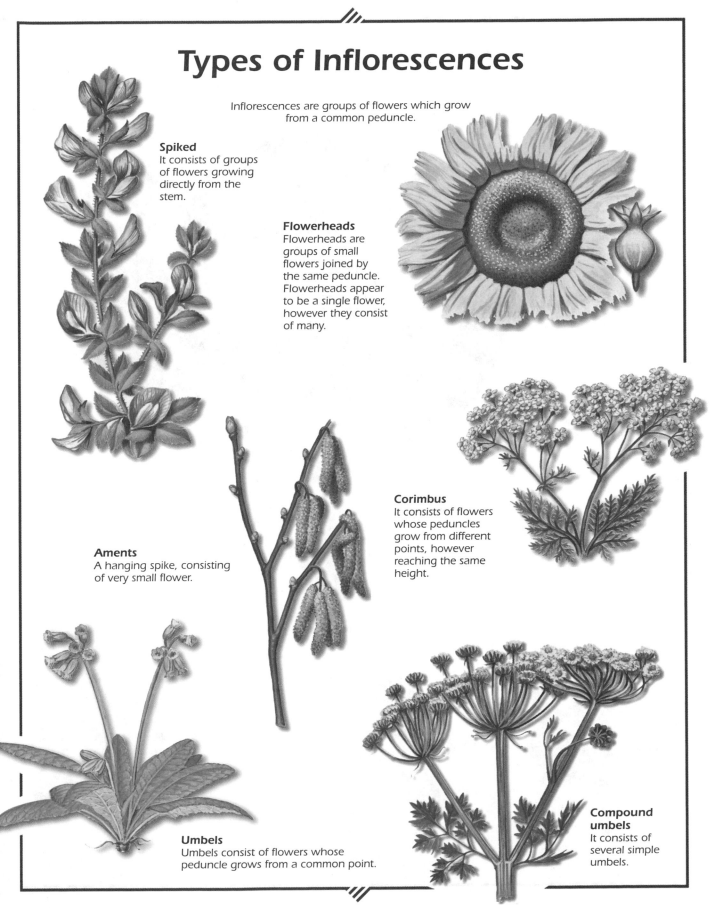

Spiked
It consists of groups
of flowers growing
directly from the
stem.

Flowerheads
Flowerheads are
groups of small
flowers joined by
the same peduncle.
Flowerheads appear
to be a single flower,
however they consist
of many.

Corimbus
It consists of flowers
whose peduncles
grow from different
points, however
reaching the same
height.

Aments
A hanging spike, consisting
of very small flower.

Umbels
Umbels consist of flowers whose
peduncle grows from a common point.

**Compound
umbels**
It consists of
several simple
umbels.

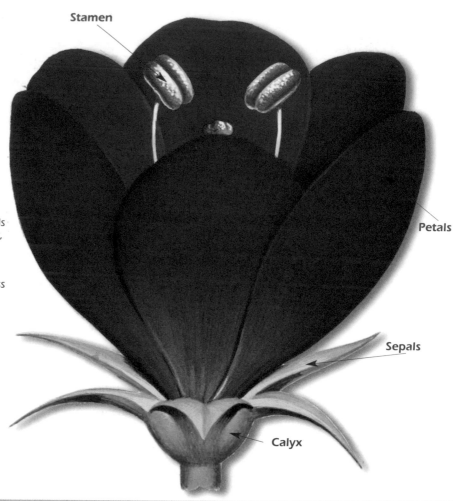

Stamen

Petals

Sepals

Calyx

The **flower** is the reproductive organ of **fanerogamous** plants (with flowers). These plants are divided into two groups: **gymnosperms,** whose seeds are uncovered (with no fruit, such as the pine tree and other Coniferae) and **angiosperms,** whose seeds are covered by a more or less fleshy fruit. The flowers of angiosperm plants are the largest and most beautiful.

Types of Flowers

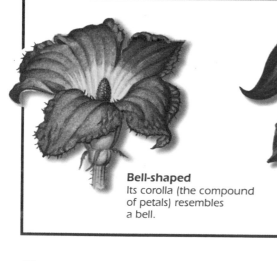

Bell-shaped
Its corolla (the compound of petals) resembles a bell.

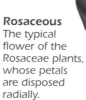

Lip-shaped
The petals form two lips, an upper one and a lower one.

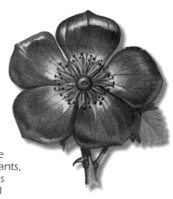

Rosaceous
The typical flower of the Rosaceae plants, whose petals are disposed radially.

# of a Flower

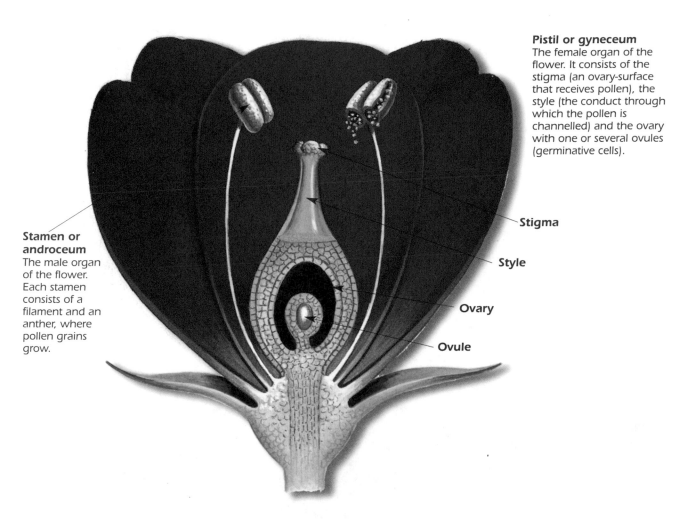

Pistil or gyneceum
The female organ of the flower. It consists of the stigma (an ovary-surface that receives pollen), the style (the conduct through which the pollen is channelled) and the ovary with one or several ovules (germinative cells).

—— Stigma

—— Style

—— Ovary

—— Ovule

Stamen or androceum
The male organ of the flower. Each stamen consists of a filament and an anther, where pollen grains grow.

A Grain of Pollen

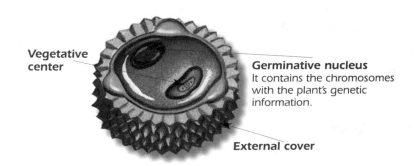

Vegetative center

Germinative nucleus
It contains the chromosomes with the plant's genetic information.

External cover

The fecundation of flowers
In order for fecundation (fertilization) to take place, to form the seed and then the fruit, a grain of pollen must Fall on the stigma of the flower. When the pollen and the flower belong to the same species, the pollen produces an elongation which goes down the style to the ovary. There, the male pollen chromosomes join the female ovule chromosomes, thus forming the seed and the fruit.
Plants with flowers reproduce sexually. This means that there are two parts, male or female, which must join to give birth to a new plant.

Guardians or Killers?
Endangered Plants

Plants are **indispensable** life agents of the Earth. All animals and human beings depend on green plants for food, because plants are **the only** living beings able to take advantage of solar energy and which produce carbohydrates, proteins, fats, vitamins and other organic substances.

Plants make decisive contributions to the **ecological balance** and to the preservation of the **environment.** They prevent soil erosion, store water and fertilize the ground.

Plants are a very important source of medicinal substances.

Each one of the 390,000-odd vegetal species living on the Earth is a different living form, with its own, unique genes. When any species disappears or becomes extinct, there is an irreparable loss in mankind's biological heritage.

Human beings, who should be the guardians of this biodiverse legacy conferred upon us by the Creator, often become its killers. According to the International Union for Nature Preservation, 20% of the 390,000 species all over the world (some 78,000) are endangered and may disappear. The Smithsonian Institution of the United States calculates that out of the 20,000 different seed or flowering species living on the continent of the United States, ten percent (some 2,000) have already disappeared, are endangered, or at risk.

What are the causes of such vegetal species disappearing? According to the *Red Book of Endangered Vegetal Species*, published by the Ministry of Agriculture of Spain, these are some of them:

- Forest **fires.**

- **Tourist development** of coasts and mountain lands.

- Water, soil and air **pollution** (because of farm herbicides).

"Forests appear before civilizations. Deserts follow civilizations."
François-René Chateaubriand (1768-1848), French author and politician.

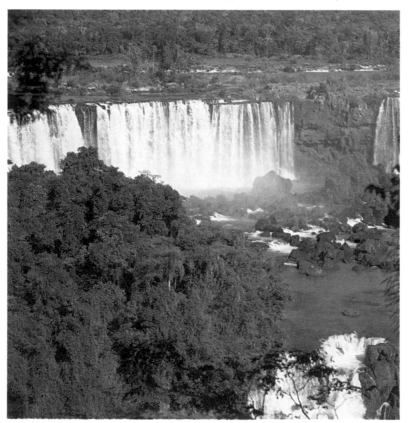

Gathering, not Plundering

- *Gather only in those **places** where this practice is **allowed,** never in natural or national parks, nor in biological reserves.*

- ***Respect protected species,** for they are endangered (get information from the agriculture authorities of the area first).*

- *Gather only **small amounts** of plants, especially when they are not abundant.*

- *Gather, but do **not kill or uproot** the plants if possible.*

When we maintain and protect the plants of our planet, we are helping to cure and alleviate many present and future illnesses, among other things.

- Amateurs **gathering** rare species.
- **Building** of dams, highways and roads.

Could we imagine how significant the loss of the *Cinchona* trees in South American forests would have been, if they had been razed by bulldozers before quinine, which prevents malaria, was discovered? What if those beautiful flowers of the foxglove family had been prematurely gathered before the heart-stimulant glycosides which have healed so many people with heart disease had been discovered?

Let us *all* do our part to preserve vegetal species in the best way. And if we go out gathering plants, let us bear in mind the advice for gathering, not plundering.

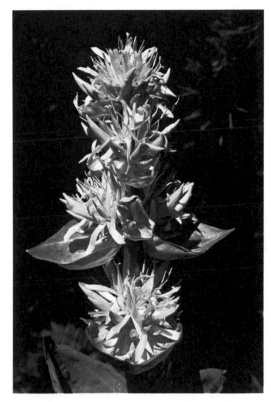

The picture on the left shows the fantastic Iguazu Falls, on the border between Brazil and Argentina. South America houses the largest forests on the planet, a true vegetal reserve which hides many botanical-medicinal secrets. This is why the Amazon forest has been called "the largest pharmacy in the world."

Gentian ("Gentiana lutea" L.) is one of many endangered plants, so it never must be picked.

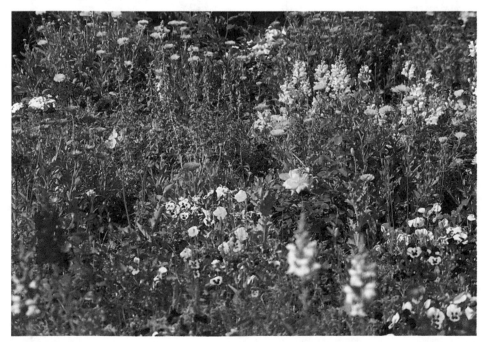

According to the Holy Bible, plants were the first to be created and could thus exist without animals and human beings. However, animals and human beings could never survive without plants. To respect and protect them is one of our duties as inhabitants of the Earth.

Photosynthesis
The Chemical Basis of Life on Earth

Photosynthesis takes place in two phases:

First phase:

$$6\ H_2O + 6\ CO_2 \longrightarrow C_6H_{12}O_6 + 6\ O_2$$

Water + Carbon dioxide = Glucose + Oxygen

Second phase:

$$n\ (C_6H_{12}O_6) \longrightarrow n\ (C_6H_{10}O_5) + n\ (H_2O)$$

Several glucose molecules together = Starch + Several water molecules

From two inorganic substances, water (which plants absorb from the soil) and carbon dioxide (a gas which is absorbed from the atmosphere), plants produce first glucose and then starch, two organic substances that are part of living beings. From the glucose, the mineral nitrogen, and other soil elements, vegetables produce all substances that form them through a complex series of chemical reactions.

This formidable chemical reaction, photosynthesis, is possible only due to chlorophyll, a green pigment which is only found in green plants and acts as the catalyst for the reaction.

Photosynthesis is the chemical basis of life on earth, and though it seems quite simple, it has never been reproduced in a laboratory by any means. Thanks to photosynthesis, simple elements become complex: inorganic substances become organic substances. In other words: dead elements—from the soil and the atmosphere—are transformed into living compounds—vegetables.

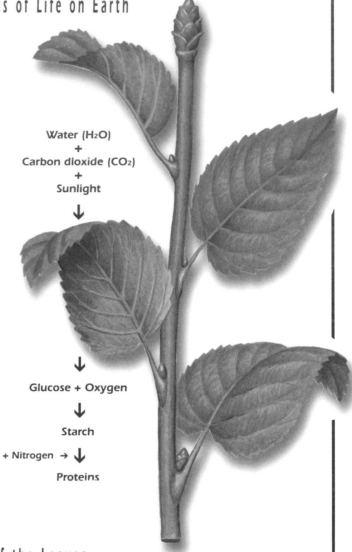

Water (H_2O)
+
Carbon dioxide (CO_2)
+
Sunlight
↓

↓

Glucose + Oxygen
↓
Starch
+ Nitrogen → ↓
Proteins

Functions of the Leaves

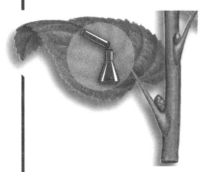

1. Production of sap from the substances absorbed by the root.

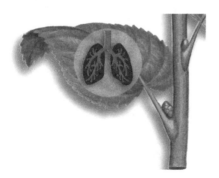

2. Production of oxygen and water vapor, as result of photosynthesis.

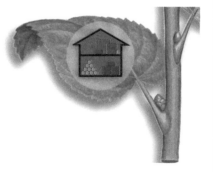

3. Storage of nutrients such as starch, sugars, vitamins, etc.

Methods for Distilling Essences

• **Distillation:** It is done by means of a device called a still. The water inside the still is heated to boiling point. The volatile active ingredients of the plants which lie over the water are carried by the water vapor. That vapor, which contains the active principles of the plants, passes through a refrigerating circuit where it cools and condenses, forming a liquid. Once the process has ended, when steeping the distilled liquid, two fractions are separated by decanting the liquid into:

- **essential oil** (essence), which forms the upper layer because of its low density, and its insolubility in water, and;

- **floral water** (hydrosol), which is the condensed water vapor, along with the watersoluble substances it has carried. There are also small amounts of essential oils present in suspension in the flower water. Floral waters are used mainly to make perfumes, although research is currently examining their medicinal applications.

• **Expression:** The application of pressure on the active parts of the plant until the essence is extracted. This method is especially used to obtain the essences of citrus rind (orange, lemon and tangerine).

• **Extraction with solvents:** The aromatic elements of plants are dissolved into a volatile solvent, which is later evaporated, leaving a dry residue called **absolute essence.**

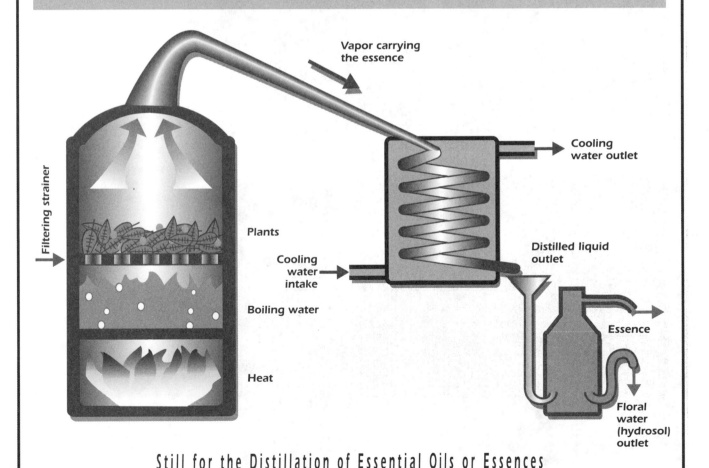

Vapor carrying the essence

Cooling water outlet

Filtering strainer

Plants

Cooling water intake

Boiling water

Heat

Distilled liquid outlet

Essence

Floral water (hydrosol) outlet

Still for the Distillation of Essential Oils or Essences

The Art of Preparing Herbal Teas

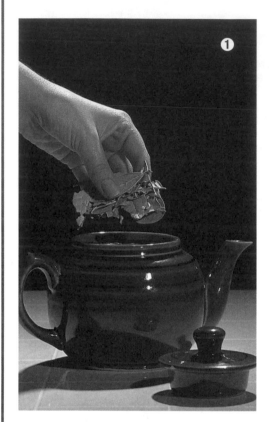

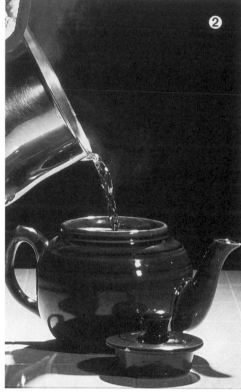

1. Put the part of the plant to be used in an suitable container. The plants may be loose or placed into a tea strainer or a small bag. The usual method is to first introduce the plants, and then pour water over them, but this can also be done the other way round.

2. Blanch the plants with almost boiling water.

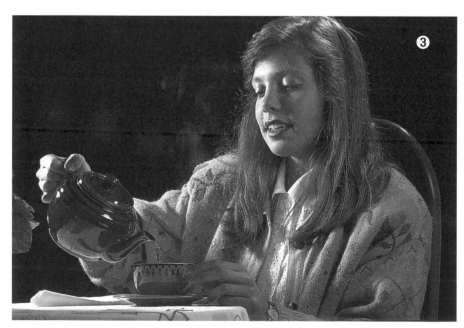

3. Drink the infusion after letting it steep and cool in a covered container to avoid loss of active ingredients through evaporation.

Fomentations
Method of Application

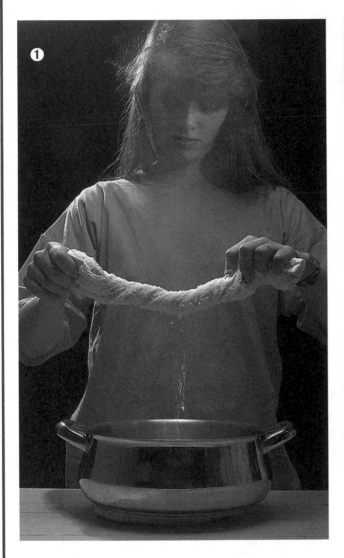

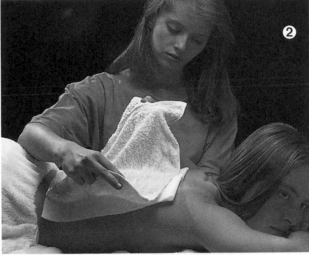

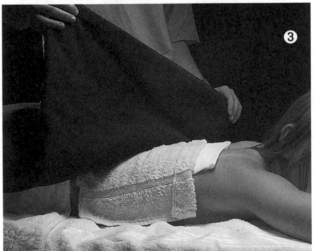

1. Prepare one or two liters of **infusion or decoction** of the plant. It is usually better if they are slightly **more concentrated** than usual (50 to 100 g per liter of water). From five to ten drops of **essence** of the plant may be also added to one or two liters of hot water.

2. When the liquid is **hot,** soak a **cotton cloth or towel** (picture ❶).

3. **Wring** out the cloth, then apply it to the affected area, protecting the skin with **another dry cloth** (picture ❷).

4. **Cover** these two cloths with a **woollenblanket** to maintain the heat. Wool preserves heat better, even when wet or soaked (picture ❸). Care should be taken that the person is not burned.

5. After **three minutes**, when the cloth begins to cool, soak it again in the hot liquid.

6. The application of fomentations must take place for **15 to 20 minutes.** To finish, **rub cold water** on the affected area.

Safe Use of Medicinal Herbs

The first step is to adopt a healthy lifestyle

Before applying any plant regularly or continuously (as with any other medicine), one must bear in mind the following points:

1. **Look for the causes of the disease,** even when symptoms seem to lack significance. Taking any plant (as with any other medicine) with the sole aim of easing or neutralizing certain symptoms may merely produce a temporary healing.

However, when the cause of the symptoms is not attacked, the disease will continue to develop until it appears with greater intensity, and then it may be too late to cure it.

When a strange symptom appears, it is better to ask for a *professional medical diagnosis* to be carried out, with *scientific* means and procedures. Only after that can a medicinal herb based treatment or any other cure be safely applied.

2. **Give up bad health habits.** When disorders or symptoms are due to unhealthy habits, or to an unhealthy lifestyle, treatment with plants will be less than useless, and it even may be harmful by masking certain symptoms while their cause develops.

The **first step** to restoring health should be the adoption of a **healthy lifestyle,** and the avoidance of bad habits. Taking mucolythic or expectorant plants to heal bronchitis is useless if a person continues smoking or breathing polluted air.

Most of the chronic diseases in developed countries are directly related to poor eating habits and the consumption of toxic substances such as tobacco, alcoholic beverages, and other drugs.

3. **Use only well-identified plants.** It is recommended and safest to make sure that plants are bottled and correctly labelled under the auspices of a pharmaceutical laboratory or professional.

The laws of many countries, including the European Union, forbid the sale of medicinal herbs by peddlers.

4. **Avoid self-prescriptions.** It is best that plants are prescribed or recommended by a competent physician.

Notwithstanding, the health laws of most countries list certain plants which may be freely used without a medical prescription. In this case, we recommend **responsible self-prescription:** one decides which plants are going to be taken, but in a responsible way. First, educate yourself on the properties of the plants as well as the precautions that their use requires.

5. **Be cautious when taking a plant for long periods of time.** As a rule, avoid the continuous use of any plant for more than two or three months. When the condition seems to require this, it is better to be informed on possible undesirable side effects of the plant. Requesting medical counsel is also advised.

6. **Care must be taken with pregnant women and with children.** As with all medicines, extreme caution is required when any medicinal herb is to be given to pregnant women and children (see pages 101-102).

Practical Cases

An adequate use of medicinal herbs, as well as the adoption of healthy life style habits may prevent weakness of our bodies from evolving into open diseases.

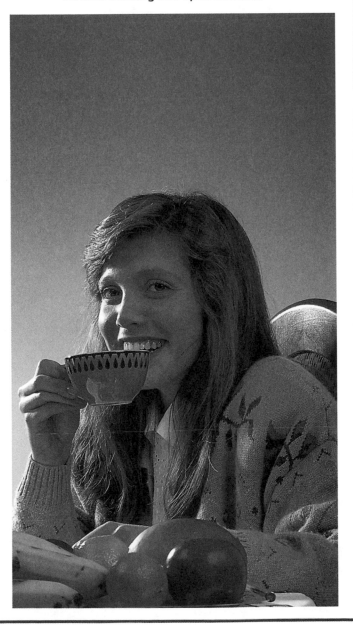

1. Look for the cause of the illness

John was a robust man, aged 55, who had never suffered serious illness. More than a year ago, he lost his appetite, and certain foods, such as meat, made him nauseous.

He prescribed for himself some plants that a neighbor recommended. He was assured they were quite effective in the recovery of appetite. During the first months he improved. However later, though he had no pain, his appetite did not improve, and he lost weight. Finally he decided to see a doctor.

An endoscopic exam of his intestine revealed that the cause of his lack of appetite was stomach cancer. The tumor was too large for successful surgical results.

This is a typical case of stomach cancer. Had John consulted the cause of his symptoms when they appeared, the prognostic of his disease would have been more favorable.

2. Avoid bad health habits

Steve was a truck-driver, who spent many hours driving. He suffered from hemorrhoids, which quite often became swollen and bled.

Steve liked spicy foods with chili and pepper. He seldom ate fruit. When he ate spicy meals, he noticed that his 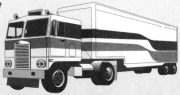 hemorrhoids worsened. He discovered some plants recommended at a natural remedy store. Using them in hip baths, he obtained much relief. He continued eating spicy meals and taking hip baths.

Nonetheless, the hemorrhoids worsened and one day he felt an intense pain which neither the plants nor any other remedy could alleviate. His doctor sent him to a surgeon: the diagnosis was hemorrhoid thrombosis, a very painful complication of hemorrhoids.

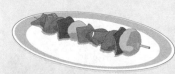

Had Steve adopted healthier eating habits, his hemorrhoids would not have worsened, and the medicinal hip baths he used would have been enough to improve and even heal his ailment.

Aromatherapy (1)
The Therapeutical Use of Essential Oils (Essences)

The Power of Aroma

Before reaching the lungs and passing into the blood, the molecules of the essence stimulate the olfactory (smell) cells in the **nostrils** [1].

These cells are actually neurons, which through the olfactory nerve send electric pulses with the coded smelling message. The **smell nerve** [2] carries the stimulus to different parts of the brain: the amygdala and the hippocampus of the **temporal lobe** [3], where scent memory lies; the **thalamus** [4], where emotions lie, and overall, the **hypothalamus** [5], and, through-out it, the **hypophysis** [6], the regulating center of hormone production for the whole body.

The relationship between the olfactory nerve, the thalamus, the hypothalamus, and the hypophysis could explain the well-known regulative effects of aromas on the neuro-hormonal system.

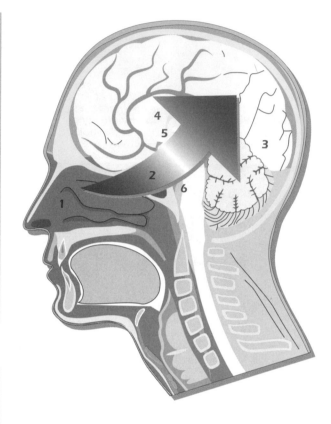

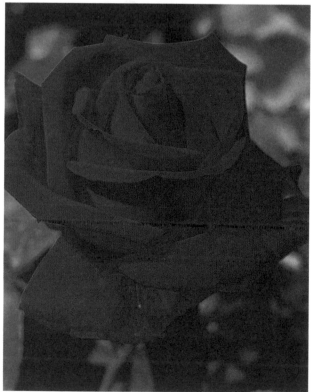

Aromatherapy, which literally means "treatment by means of aromas," is actually one of the methods of phytotherapy ("treatment by means of plants"). The healing properties of essential oils were known in ancient times, though only in an empirical way. Today, we know the reason why essential oils produce certain physiological effects on the body. However, there is much research still needed on how certain aromas influence the state of mind and even behavior.

In order to obtain good results, treatment with essential oils must last from one to three weeks, applied in any of the following four ways:

1. **atmospheric diffusion**
2. **massaging the skin**
3. **essence baths**
4. **internal use**

1. Atmospheric Diffusion

This is the most important way to take advantage of the healing properties of essential oils. These can pass into the air in several ways:

- By simple **evaporation,** by putting some drops on the back of the hand or over a **heat source,** such as a heater, and smelling the aroma. Also, a handkerchief or even a pillow may be impregnated with some drops of essence.

- By means of an **electric diffuser,** a small device which uses a vibrating mechanism to produce **vaporization** of the essential oil it contains. It has the advantage of working without heat, then the essence turns into vapor without undergoing the undesirable effects of heat. Ten to fifteen minutes of work are enough to fill a room with microparticles of vaporized essences.

(continued on next page)

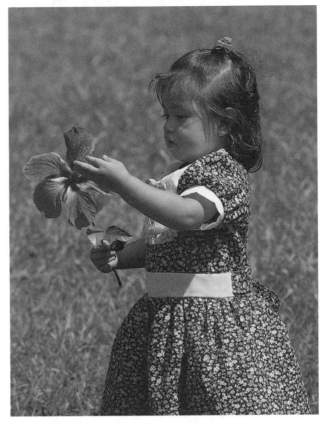

The simple act of smelling the aroma of a flower affects the hormonal balance, the nervous system, the respiratory system, and even our state of mind.

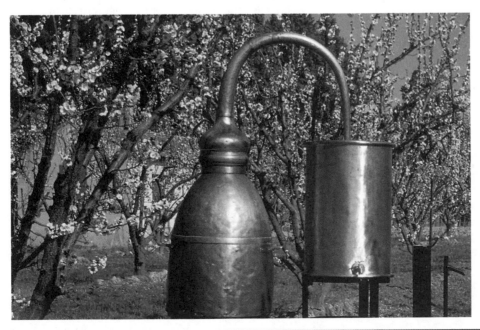

Essential oils are mainly obtained by means of distillation in stills, as in the picture, which belongs to the Aroma and Perfume Museum (La Chevêche de Graveson-en-Provence, France).

In order to produce a good essence, certain degrees of art and patience are required. From one hundred kg of eucalyptus leaves, for instance, only two liters of essential oil are obtained.

Aromatherapy (2)

Create Your Own Environment Using Essences

It is better to use **only one essential oil** at a time instead of mixing several of them.

Depending on the desired effects, some environments may be created with one of the following essences:

- **Balsamic** environment for cases of sinusitis, laryngitis and certain respiratory diseases, with essence of eucalyptus, pine tree, thyme, or rosemary.
- **Relaxed and sedative** environment, for nervousness or insomnia, with essence of English lavender or orange. Both essences are especially recommended for nervous children who do not Fall asleep easily.
- **Stimulating** environment, with the essence of lemon, rosemary, peppermint or Winter savory.
- **Antiseptic** environment to prevent contagion in the case of influenza or colds, with essence of thyme, sage, eucalyptus, or cinnamon.
- An environment to **repel mosquitos** and other insects, with essence of balm or lemon verbena.
- **Anti-tobacco** environment, with the essence of lemon verbena, geranium, sassafras or English lavender.

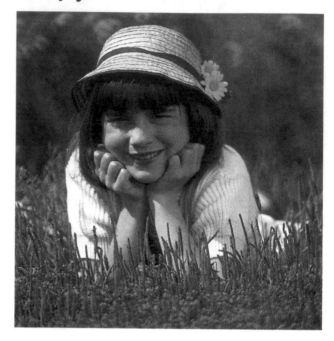

(continued from previous page)

2. Topical Application

Rubbing essential oil on the skin makes it penetrate, soaking the tissues and passing finally to the blood and lymphatic system. The proper effect of the essential oil is enhanced by rubbing, which is when the results are notable. When essential oils are applied by friction to the skin, the following points should be remembered:

- **Massage** the chest, the stomach, the back, the neck, the arms, and the legs.
- **Avoid any contact** of the essential oil with the mucosa of eyes, mouth, and genitals.
- For normal application, **20 to 30 drops** of essential oil are enough. The oil must be applied to the hands of the person rubbing.
- In the case of **sensitive skin,** the essence may be **diluted** by mixing it 50/50 with olive, wheat germ, or bitter almond oil.

Massage Using Essences

Depending on the desired effect, massage using one of the following essential oils:

- **Stimulating** massage, preferably in the morning, after a cold shower, with essence of rosemary, geranium, lemon or pine tree.
- **Relaxing** massage, applied at night after a hot shower or bath, with essence of English lavender, marjoram, camomile or orange.
- **Digestive** massage, applied to the stomach after every meal in order to avoid gases and digestive problems, with caraway, marjoram, or English lavender oil.
- **Respiratory** massage, applied to the chest and back, and recommendable in case of colds, bronchitis, asthma, and cold coughs, with essence of pine tree, eucalyptus, English lavender, rosemary or cypress.
- **Analgesic** massage, on the legs or the back, to alleviate muscular or joint aches, with essence of rosemary, juniper, pine tree or marjoram.
- **Circulatory** massage, to improve the return of venous blood in the case of varicose veins, swollen legs, or cellulitis, with essence of cypress or lemon.

Besides producing a pleasant sensation of well-being, the inhalation of essences (aromatotherapy) may exert notable medicinal actions: restore sleep in cases of insomnia, balance the nervous system when dealing with depression or fatigue, increase breathing capacity, and normalize blood pressure, among other things.

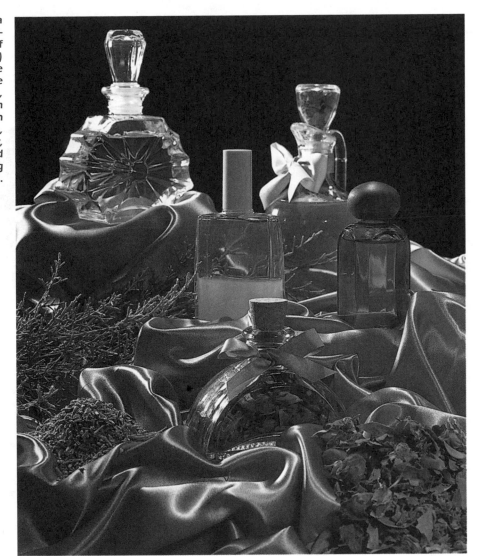

3. Baths with Essences

The essential oils mentioned in previous treatments may be also added to bath water. Three to ten drops per bathtub are used.

Essences are also added to the water of vapor inhalations. In this case, two or three drops are enough.

4. Internal Use

Though it is not the ideal method of application, essential oils may be also taken orally as a complement to any of the previous treatments. The same essence used for diffusion, massage, or baths may be taken to reinforce its effect, but it should be noted that:

• Essential oils are highly concentrated active principles, consequently **their doses must not be exceeded.** Generally these doses are one to three drops, three or four times a day.

• Never take an essential oil for **more than three weeks.**

• **Children under six** should not take essential oils. They should rather take hydrosols.

• Essential oils should be taken in any of the following ways:

– Pouring drops on the back of the **hand.**

– Pouring them on a spoon **with honey.**

– Pouring them into a glass with **lukewarm water** (never hot water, because the active components decompose with heat).

Abortive Plants

Warning: None of the so called abortive plants suffice to produce an abortion. There is an old sentence attributed to Hippocrates which reads: "There are no abortive substances, but those which are toxic for both the mother and the fetus."

Provoking an abortion with any of these plants requires such a high dose that they will surely cause intoxication in the mother with severe undesirable effects such as intestinal colics, vomiting, nervous excitation, convulsions, etc. There have been cases of pregnant women who have died when trying to produce an abortion with plants.

When we point out "abortion risk" in the table of plants to avoid during pregnancy (p. 43) we do not mean the plant is abortive in absolute terms, but that it increases the risk of an abortion in women who are already predisposed to it because of any other reason, known or unknown.

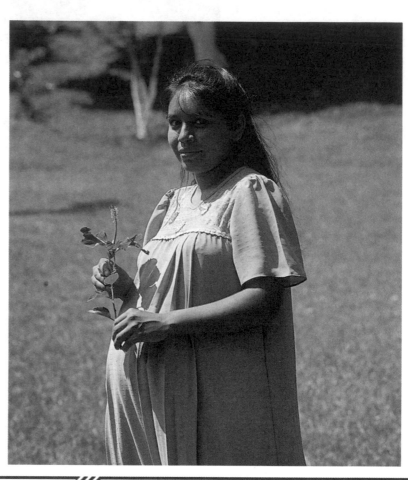

Trying to produce an abortion with toxic plants puts the mother, as well as the fetus, at a severe risk of death.

The Importance of Correct Dosage

*For **toxic plants** (such as foxglove) the **toxic dose** is **very close to the therapeutic dose,** thus the margin of safety is very narrow. A **double** dose of that recommended as therapeutic may provoke **toxic effects**, and a **triple** dose may cause **death.***
*However, in **non-toxic plants** (such as thyme) one can take **ten times the recommended dose** without suffering significant symptoms, as there is no fatal dose: no matter what the amount of plant is taken, as **there is no risk** of it causing poisoning.*

Plant	Used part	Therapeutic dose	Toxic dose	Deadly dose
Foxglove (example of **toxic** plant)	Dried leaves powder	1 g (daily)	2 g (vomiting, bradycardia, diarrhea)	3 g (cold sweat, convulsions, arrhythmias of the heart, heart failure)
Thyme (example of **non-toxic** plant)	Flower clusters	20 g (daily)	200 g (minor symptoms: excitation, nausea)	None

Plants to Avoid During Pregnancy

Sage

During pregnancy all toxic plants, as well as the following, must be avoided.

Plant	Reason
Alder buckthorn	Laxative/purgative, produces pelvic congestion
Aloe	Oxytocic, produces uterine contractions
Boldo	Not proven, but it can affect the fetus
Boxwood	Can produce vomiting and nervous irritation
Cascara sagrada	Laxative/purgative, produces pelvic congestion
Coffee tree	Decreases fetal growth
Fraxinella	Emmenagogue, risk of abortion
Jalap	Purgative and emmenagogue, risk of abortion
Licorice	Produces hypertension and edema when used for long periods
Mugwort	Emmenagogue, risk of abortion
Parsley	Emmenagogue, risk of abortion
Pomegranate	Toxic alkaloids, possible fetal alteration (bark)
Rhubarb	Purgative, produces pelvic congestion
Saffron	Risk of abortion when taken in high doses
Sage	Oxytocic, contracts the uterus
Tansy	Emmenagogue (tuyone), risk of abortion
Tinnevelly senna	Purgative, produces uterine contractions
Watercress	Risk of abortion
Wormwood	Emmenagogue, risk of abortion

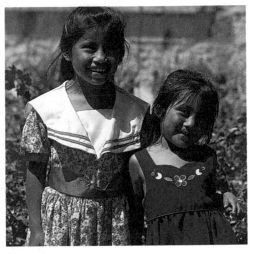

Children, like pregnant women, must be careful when using any plant or medicine.

Plant Toxicity

Accidents related to the use of diverse plants in general, and with medicinal herbs particularly, are not rare. Children mostly suffer from this kind of poisoning, which may be deadly. It is important to know how to prevent plant poisoning, and how to act when the event occurs.

Causes of Toxicity

Plant toxicity usually occurs due to:

- **mistaking** a poisonous plant for a medicinal one, or
- administering an **excessive dose** of a potentially toxic plant.

Prevention

It is better to avoid poisoning rather than treat it. In order to avoid toxic reactions one must:

1. Positively **identify** any plant before taking it. Be very careful with plants other people give us, or that of alleged botanical experts.

2. **Weigh the dose** of the plant to be administered.

3. **Watch children** when going to the countryside. Most cases of poisoning occur in children who suck or chew on flowers and plants.

4. **Never plant toxic species** in gardens, or in places where children may visit.

How To Obtain the Best Results From Plants

The best results are obtained by using plants combined with other natural agents that offer medicinal action, such as **water** (hydrotherapy), **the sea** (talasotherapy), **the sun** (heliotherapy), **medicinal soils** (geotherapy), **physical exercise** and **healthy food** based on vegetal products.

Moreover, a healthy lifestyle is required, which means **avoiding tobacco,** alcoholic beverages, and other drugs.

The **combined action** of all these factors is a notable stimulant on the defensive and health mechanisms of the body, which will finally overcome the disease.

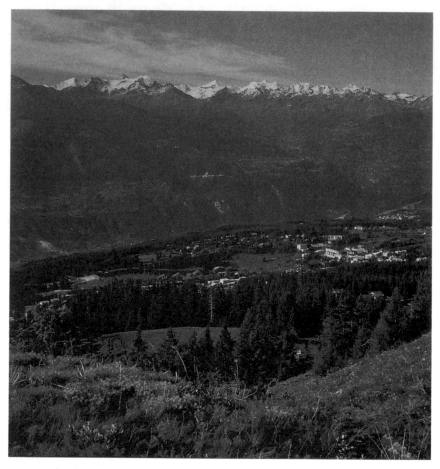

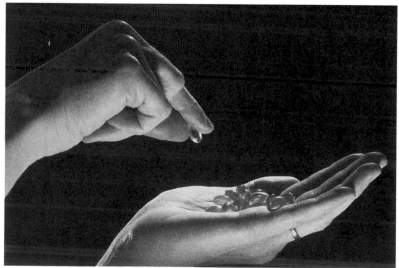

In vegetal remedies, the active components have the advantage of being combined with many other substances that appear to be inactive. However, these complementary components give the plant as a whole a safety and efficiency much superior to that of its isolated and pure active components.

Furthermore, the efficiency of medicinal herbs increases when they are used within the frame of natural revitalizing treatment.

A Pioneer of Modern Phytotherapy

In the late nineteenth and early twentieth centuries, physicians still prescribed medicines based on very energetic chemical substances, some of which were recently discovered and at present are regarded as poisonous: **calomel** or mercuric cyanide (with strongly purgative action), **tartar emetic** (vomitive), **strychnine** (toxic excitant), or **arsenic salts** (against syphilis and other infectious diseases).

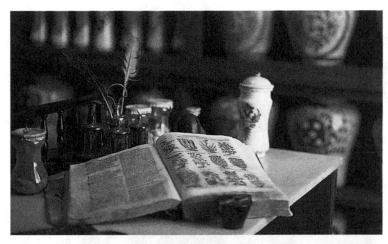

The developments of the newly-born **chemical and pharmaceutical industry,** both in Europe and in the United States, had brought about great social enthusiasm. The ongoing discovery of more and more powerful new medicines, though not less toxic, seemed to promise a near future in which there was to be a specific pharmacological product to treat every disease.

Within that environment of pharmacological euphoria, when all scientific interest was placed on chemically synthesized medicines, Ellen G. White, an outstanding American author with great teaching and preventive ability, wrote: *"There are simple herbs that can be used for the recovery of the sick, whose effect upon the system is very different from that of those drugs that poison the blood and endanger life."* *

This pioneer of modern phytotherapy recommended the popular use of certain medicinal herbs, advancing the current laws of most Western countries by more than 100 years, which allow the free use of certain plants without medical prescription, such as **hops** infusion (sedative), **foot baths with mustard** (to clear the head), **charcoal** (because of its detoxifying effect), and **pine, cedar,** and **fir trees** (for respiratory diseases).

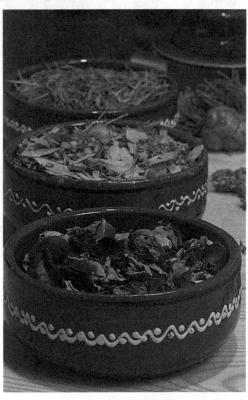

Besides promoting the rational use of medicinal herbs as an alternative to the aggressive medicinal remedies used at that time, Ellen G. White emphasized a fact currently well-known in medical science, which however was a real novelty a century ago: **Health does not come naturally,** but through a healthy way of life, and especially, from nutrition.

Today, her central idea about health is truer than ever: the intelligent use of **natural agents** such as water, the sun, air, medicinal herbs, healthy food, as well as the adoption of healthy habits (physical exercise, adequate rest, good mental health, and trust in God) may do more for health than all powerful, chemically synthesized medicines or aggressive treatments.

* *Selected Messages*, Book 2, p. 288, Review & Herald Publishing Association, Washington D.C., 1958.

The adequate use of medicinal plants, along with other healthy life style habits, may prevent our inherent body weaknesses from becoming manifested diseases.

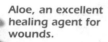

Cocoa, a stimulant, diuretic, and wound healing agent.

Aloe, an excellent healing agent for wounds.

Corn, a diuretic meal.

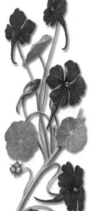

Nasturtium, an antibiotic plant.

Medicinal Herb

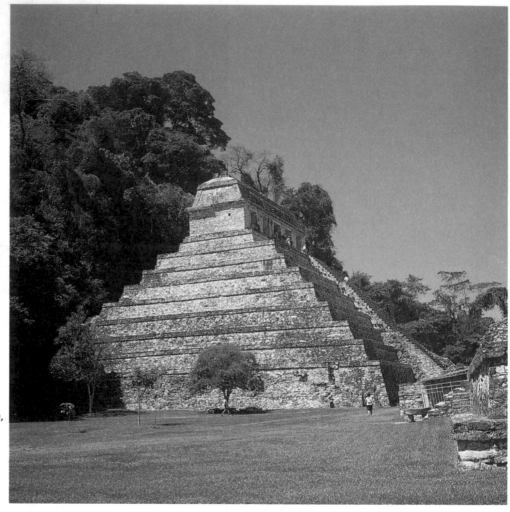

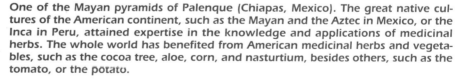

One of the Mayan pyramids of Palenque (Chiapas, Mexico). The great native cultures of the American continent, such as the Mayan and the Aztec in Mexico, or the Inca in Peru, attained expertise in the knowledge and applications of medicinal herbs. The whole world has benefited from American medicinal herbs and vegetables, such as the cocoa tree, aloe, corn, and nasturtium, besides others, such as the tomato, or the potato.

"I request Your Majesty that no more physicians are ever allowed to enter New Spain (Mexico), as there are already sufficient medicine men there."

These were the words of the Spanish conquistador Hernán Cortés to Emperor Charles, the first of Spain and the fifth of Germany, in 1522, after having been successfully treated by Aztec physicians of a head wound which Spanish physicians were not able to heal.

It is evident that native medicine men knew well how to take advantage of the rich Mexican medicinal flora, a fact which gave them a notable advantage over their Spanish colleagues.

Medical science in general, and the use of medicinal herbs in particular, were truly developed in the Aztec, Mayan and Inca cultures, as well as among the North American natives.

In **Mexico,** capital of the Anahuac region, large botanical gar-

n America

Echinacea, a natural stimulant of body defenses.

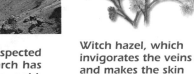

Goldenseal, quite effective against colds.

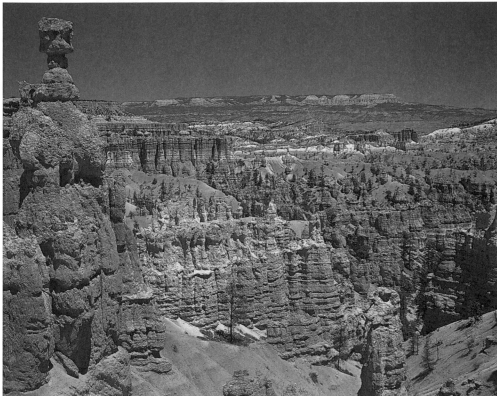

A view of the Bryce Canyon (Utah, USA). North American natives knew and respected the resources of nature, especially medicinal herbs. Modern scientific research has proved the effectiveness of many plants used by natives, such as echinacea, goldenseal, and witch hazel.

Witch hazel, which invigorates the veins and makes the skin more beautiful.

dens surrounded the Emperor's palaces, in which plants from the whole empire were grown.

Dr. José María Reverte Coma, professor of history at the Universidad Complutense of Madrid, recounts that in ancient Mexico there were different health science professionals:

• The **tlama-tepati-ticiti**, general physicians who healed with plants, baths, diets, and purgative or laxative substances.

• The **texoxo-tlacicitl**, who were expert surgeons.

• The **papiani-panamacani**, who were herb experts.

The Spanish explorers were astonished by the great diversity of new medicinal herbs—and food herbs—which the "New World" grew.

Dr. Diego Alvarez Chanca, a Spanish physician who accompanied Cortés on his first journey to America, was first to describe the potato, cocoa, corn, cassava, copaiba, guaiac, and brazilwood. Other people discovered cinchona, sarsaparilla, aloe, mandrake, rhatany, quassia, nasturtium, and many other medicinally interesting plants.

During the seventeenth and eighteenth centuries, different botanical expeditions left Europe in order to study the medicinal flora of America. Perhaps the most important of these expeditions was the one led by José Celestino Mutis in 1760. The arrival of the new medicinal herbs brought about a truly enriching revolution in the Old World therapeutics. Cinchona was to medicine what gunpowder was to war.

At present, research on the healing properties of American plants is still being conducted, based on the traditional uses that natives give to plants. The Amazon forest is an immense pharmaceutical store for mankind, many of whose resources are still unknown. This is another reason why, apart from the ecological and environmental ones, the rain forest must be preserved.

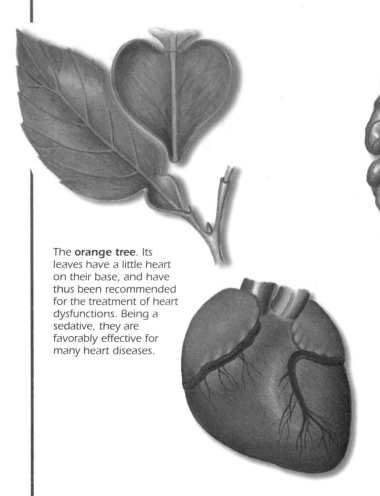

The **orange tree**. Its leaves have a little heart on their base, and have thus been recommended for the treatment of heart dysfunctions. Being a sedative, they are favorably effective for many heart diseases.

The **walnut tree**. The interior of its fruits resembles a human brain. Actually, walnuts contain phosphorus, an important element in the biochemistry of the brain and nervous system.

Ancient civilizations believed that from the features of plants they could discern their properties. This idea was already put into practice at the time of Hippocrates (fifth century B.C.): it was the so-called "theory of signs." Dioscorides himself was one of its fervent defenders. Paracelsus, a renowned Swiss physician and naturalist of the sixteenth century, said: *"Each and every vegetable is marked by nature, and to us, it is good for."*

The Theory of Signs

Like many of his contemporary colleagues, the sixteenth century Spanish physician Andrés de Laguna, who translated the *De Materia Medica* of Dioscorides into Spanish, believed that the duty of man was to discover the signs that the Creator had printed on plants as a means to decipher their virtues. Other great botanists and physicians also accepted this theory of signs during more than two thousand years. At present it seems just a historical anecdote with no scientific proof. However, it is interesting to observe how some of its propositions have been scientifically proven, for instance:

- **Walnuts** are good for the brain, because they contain considerable amounts of phosphorus and unsaturated fatty acids.

- **Birchwort** or aristolochia contains an alkaloid whose oxytocic action causes uterine contractions.

- **Sand spurry** is a diuretic plant which favors the expulsion of stones.

- **Henbane** has analgesic properties.

- **Orange tree** leaves are sedative, and are recommended for invalids.

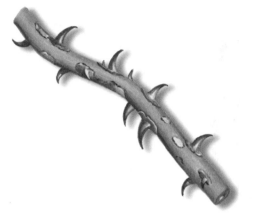

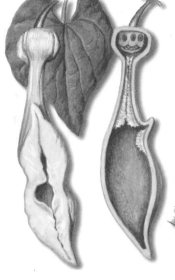

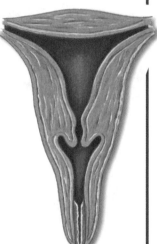

Brier hip.
Its branches resemble a dog's teeth, and thus the plant was used to heal the wounds caused by dogs' and wolves' bites. This alleged healing action has not been proven.

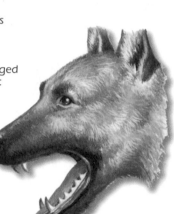

Birchwort or aristolochia.
Its flowers are similar to the female genital organs (both external and internal), thus the plant has been used to ease childbirth. We now know that the oxytocic substances it contains stimulate uterine contractions.

Of course, in many cases the theory of signs fails, in spite of being so attractive and suggestive. For instance:

- The seeds of **brier hip** do not serve in the treatment of gall stones, despite their similarity in form.

- **Clover** leaves do not cure cataracts, in spite of the white stain they have, which resembles a cataract halo.

In other cases, the allegedly deduced properties of a plant have been hyperbolized; for instance, the leaves of the **common comfrey** grow attached to its stem, and Dioscorides deduced that the plant could be a powerful wound healing agent. He was not completely wrong: the common comfrey contains alantoine, a substance which nowadays is present in many lotions. However, the enthusiastic Greek scientist affirms that the root of the common comfrey, "when cooked with chopped meat, gather and fix the meat restoring its original form."

It would not have been difficult to prove the exaggerations of Dioscorides, but ancient science was based more on conjecture than research. Thus, for many centuries, physicians recommended bathing with common comfrey water the day before marriage, for brides who wished to feign virginity when they were not virgins.

From Intuition to Experiments

Nowadays, the advanced progress in chemical and pharmaceutical research makes intuition and the tradition the theory of signs was based on unnecessary. However, the use of medicinal herbs based on superstition and sorcery, which still is alive in some social sectors, is greatly discouraged and even dangerous.

The rational and scientific use of plants, based on chemical and pharmacological research, is truly the only way to correctly use medicinal herbs.

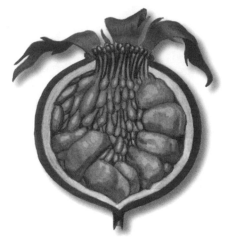

Brier hip. In the interior of its fruit there are heavy seeds which resemble gall stones. Moreover, the surface of the fruit resembles the bladder. Thus, the plant was recommended for "stone illness" (gall stones). Today, however, no scientific data is available to prove that the fruit or seeds of the brier hip are effective in fighting lithiasis.

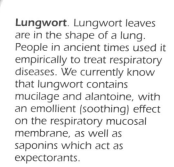

Lungwort. Lungwort leaves are in the shape of a lung. People in ancient times used it empirically to treat respiratory diseases. We currently know that lungwort contains mucilage and alantoine, with an emollient (soothing) effect on the respiratory mucosal membrane, as well as saponins which act as expectorants.

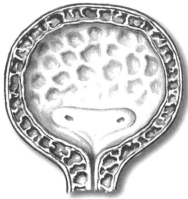

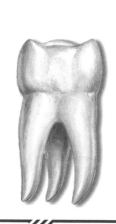

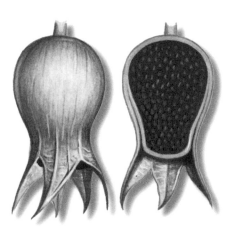

Black henbane. In ancient times, henbane was used to ease the pain of toothaches, because its fruits resemble a tooth, the calyx being the tooth roots. Today its analgesic and narcotic properties are well-known.

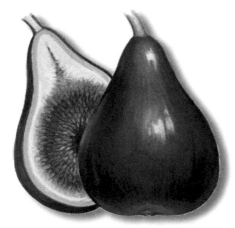

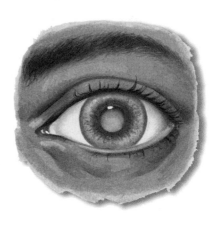

Common clover. The white stain on its leaves gave the idea that it was useful in the treatment of cataracts, but this has not been proven.

The **fig tree**. Some people have interpreted the image of hemorrhoids in figs. No experimental data has proven the effectiveness of figs on hemorrhoids.

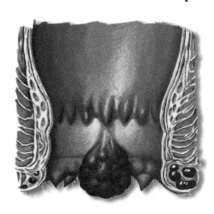

Water lily. Since it grows in cold places, its use was recommended to weaken sexual instinct (an anaphrodisiac). It is currently used for the same purpose. Besides, people who defended the theory of signs saw a symbol of virginity in its white flowers.

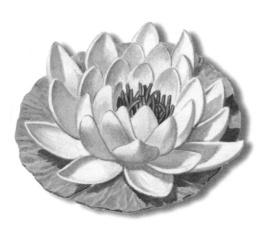

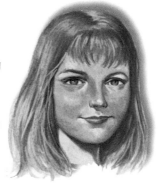

Cornflower

A good remedy for your eyes

CORNFLOWER covers the golden grain prairies from late Spring onwards with its gracious blue flowers. From ancient times, the seeds of crops have been mixed with cornflower seeds, and have been dispersed all over the world. Pliny the Elder, a first century Roman naturalist, described the cornflower as "an annoying flower for reapers," who surely tried not to cut it with their sickles and scythes. A few other words have reached us from the classical writers about this delicate plant.

Its medicinal virtues were discovered by Mattioli, a sixteenth century botanist who declared that "the blue flowers of the cornflower alleviate reddened eyes." The healing virtues of the plant were due, according to Mattioli, to the combination of opposed colors, blue versus red, in compliance with the theory of signs.

At present, herbicides and selection processes of crops are terminating with cornflower as if it were another weed.

PROPERTIES AND INDICATIONS. *FLOWERS* contain anthocyanins and polyines,

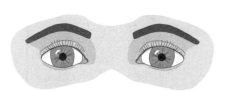

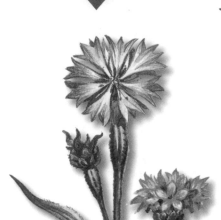

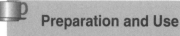

Preparation and Use

INTERNAL USE

❶ **Infusion.** 20-30 g of young flowers per liter of water. Have one cup before each meal.

EXTERNAL USE

Cornflower water. In order to obtain it, preferably fresh flowers are decocted in a proportion of 30 g (2 tablespoons) per liter of water. Boil for five minutes. It is applied on eyes when warm, in one of the following ways:

❷ **Compresses.** Soak a gauze and maintain it for 15 minutes over the affected eye, twice or three times a day.

❸ **Eye bath.** In an suitable container, or simply wringing out a soaked cloth over the affected eye. Cornflower water must fall from the temple to the nose.

❹ **Eye drops.** A few drops of cornflower water into the eye, three times a day.

Synonyms. Bluebottle, cyani, bachelor's button, bluebonnet, blue centaury.
French. Bleuet
Spanish. Azulejo, aciano, ojeras.

Habitat. It mostly grows in crop fields all over Europe, though it has reached America as well. It is less frequent in the southeastern regions of Europe.

Description. The plant belongs to the family of the Compositae. It has a thin, stiff stem, which grows up to 50 cm high. It has composite, bright blue-colored flowers, and narrow leaves which appear to be covered with a smooth velvet layer.

Parts used. Flowers.

Cornflower flowers contain anthocyanins, which have antiseptic and anti-inflammatory action. Their infusion produces an improvement in the blood circulation in the retinal capillaries, besides having appetizing and eupeptic effects.

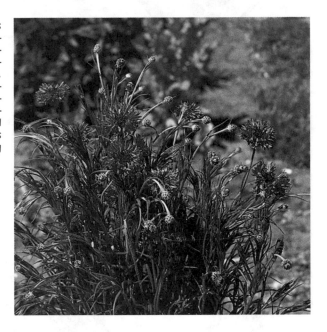

many places this plant is given the name of "bags-under-eyes." People who wash their eyes with cornflower water obtain a limpid and shimmering gaze, which flashes just like the cornflower's little blue flowers in golden wheat fields.

These are the most important indications of cornflower water.

• **Conjunctivitis** (inflammation of the mucous membrane that covers the anterior part of eyes) [❷,❸,❹]. Eye cleansing with cornflower water, as well as eye drops, will help to eliminate eye secretions (sleep) and to make eye congestion disappear.

• **Blepharitis** (inflammation of the eyelids) and **styes** (little furuncles which appear in the edge of the eyelids) [❷,❸]. In this case, the application of cornflower water in compresses or in eye baths is recommended.

In ancient times, the cornflower was supposed to clear and preserve vision, although only that of blue-eyed people. Thus, in French this plant is called *casselunettes* (glasses-breaker). Today we know that this was merely a myth, nevertheless we should remember that cornflower is good for the eyes.

whose action is **antiseptic** and **anti-inflammatory,** bitter substances which act as **appetizers** and **eupeptics** (that facilitate digestion), and also flavonoids that have a mild **diuretic** effect.

Flowers should be taken in infusions before meals [❶]. It is better not to sweeten the infusions.

CORNFLOWER WATER, obtained by the decoction of its flowers, is primarily used in applications on the eyelids, due to its notable **anti-inflammatory** effect.

Eye irrigation and baths with cornflower water ease itching and eye irritation, besides giving a fresh and smooth look to tired eyelids. Thus, in

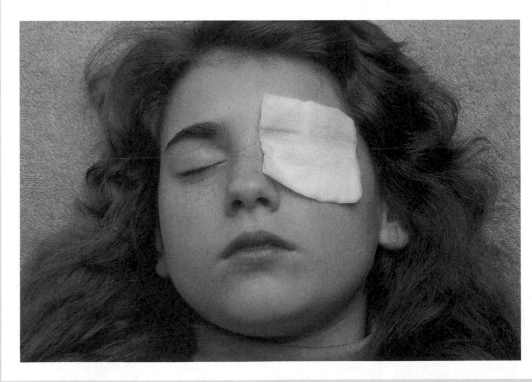

Compresses with cornflower water on the eyes reduce eyelid weariness and give a clear and shiny gaze to those who use them.

Passion Flower

An American anti-stress plant

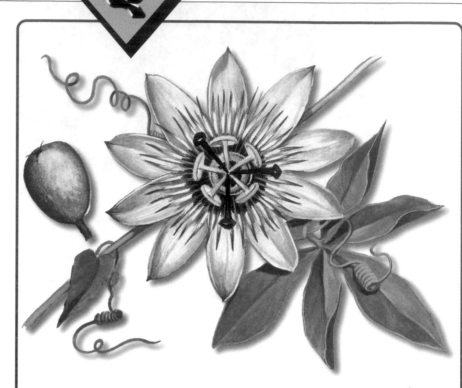

Synonyms. *Maypops, passion vine.*
French. *Passiflore, fleur de la passion.*
Spanish. *Pasionaria, granadilla, maracuyá.*

Habitat. *Native to the southern United States and Mexico, it is widespread in the tropical regions of Central and South America, mainly in the West Indies and Brazil. It grows on dry, protected areas. Naturalized in southern European Mediterranean countries.*

Description. *A woody-stem vine of the Passifloraceae family, with beautiful white or red flowers, divided into three lobes. The fruit is oval, fleshy, orange-colored, and its seeds are black.*

Parts used. *Flowers, leaves and fruits.*

THIS PLANT attracted the attention of European travellers to the New World, who saw in the diverse organs of its beautiful flowers the representation of the instruments used in the Crucifixion: whip, nails and hammer. The plant was introduced in Europe and grown as an ornamental vine, until in the late nineteenth century it was found to have a strong sedative effect on the nervous system.

PROPERTIES AND INDICATIONS. The **FLOWERS** and **LEAVES** of maypops (another name for this plant) contain small amounts of indole alkaloids, flavonoids, diverse steroids and pectin. It is not well known to which of these substances the plant owes its **sedative, antispasmodic and narcotic** (inductive of sleepiness) actions, though it is likely due to the combination of them all. Its main indications are:

• **Anxiety, nervousness, stress [❶].** The passion flower acts as a mild anxiolytic, without the risk of addiction or dependence. It is the **ideal plant** for those people who are under nervous **pressure.** The *Larousse Dictionary of Healing Plants* states that: "A gift which comes from the ancient Aztec empire, the passion flower seems to be the most necessary plant in our civilization."

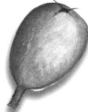

Preparation and Use

INTERNAL USE

❶ **Infusion.** The ideal way to take passion flower is with an infusion of flowers and leaves, prepared with 20-30 g per liter of water, left to rest for two or three minutes before drinking. Two or three cups daily are recommended, if desired they may be honey-sweetened. One more may be taken before bedtime in the case of insomnia.

❷ In **alcohol or drug-withdrawal treatment** the infusion is more concentrated (up to 100 g per liter), sweetened with honey. The dose depends on the patient's requirements.

• **Insomnia [❶].** The plant induces natural sleep, without drowsiness or depression on waking up. It may be administered to children, given its lack of toxicity.

• **Diverse aches and spasms [❶].** Passion flower relaxes the hollow abdominal hollow organs whose sudden contractions provoke colics or spasms: stomach, intestines (intestinal colic), bile ducts and gall bladder (liver colics), urinary ducts (kidney colic) and uterus (dysmenorrhea). The use of the passion flower is recommended for virtually any kind of pain, even neuralgia.

• **Epilepsy [❶].** As a *complementary treatment,* passion flower helps diminish the frequency and intensity of epileptic crises.

• **Alcoholism and drug-addiction [❷].** Some interesting experiments have been conducted by administering passion flower during the first days of alcohol, heroin and other drug rehabilitation treatments. This plant makes the withdrawal symptoms (the so-called "cold turkey") more easily tolerated and with less physical consequences on the body. Its sedative action allows better endurance for drug consumption on alcoholics and drug addicts, thus overcoming the anxiety of abstinence. In these cases, the plant must be used *under medical supervision.*

The *FRUITS* of the passion flower (passionfruit) are rich in provitamin A, vitamin C and organic acids. They are **refreshing and invigorating,** and are highly recommended for physical tiredness, infectious diseases, and febrile convalescence.

Purple Passion Flower

In Brazil and the West Indies another species of Passiflora *grows, the* Passiflora edulis *Sims. (=* Passiflora laurifolia *F. Vill.), which is a purple passion flower, with purple flowers (as its name indicates), also known as passionfruit. It is the best known species of the genus* Passiflora *in America.*

Purple passion flower renders a sweet, somewhat acid fruit, whose truly "tropical" flavor is present in soft drinks made with its gelatinous flesh. The oil obtained from its seeds is edible. However, **it is not considered** *to be* **a true medicinal herb.**

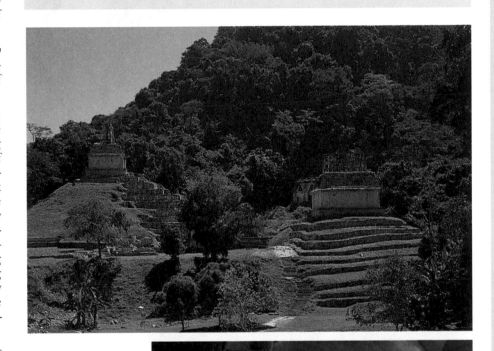

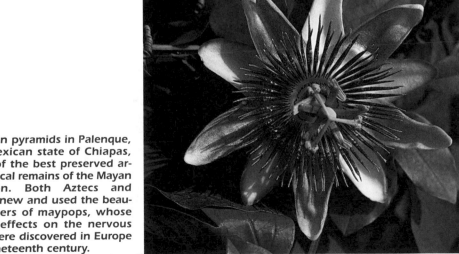

The Mayan pyramids in Palenque, in the Mexican state of Chiapas, are one of the best preserved archaeological remains of the Mayan civilization. Both Aztecs and Mayans knew and used the beautiful flowers of maypops, whose sedative effects on the nervous system were discovered in Europe in the nineteenth century.

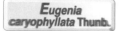

Clove Tree

Stimulant, disinfectant, and analgesic

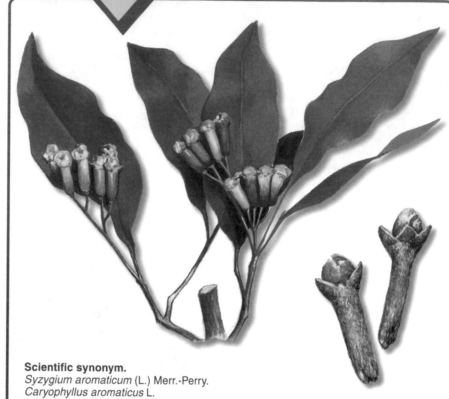

Scientific synonym.
Syzygium aromaticum (L.) Merr.-Perry.
Caryophyllus aromaticus L.

French. *Giroflier, bois a clous.*
Spanish. *Clavero, clavo de olor.*

Habitat. *Native to the Moluccas and the Philippines, at present it is grown in other tropical areas of Asia and America.*

Description. *Tree of the Mirthaceae family, growing from 10 to 20 meters high. The cloves are the flower buds, gathered when becoming red. After drying them under the sun, they acquire an ochre color.*

Parts used. *Dried flower buds.*

"COULD YOU give me a clove so that I can put it in my mouth?," a messenger coming from the Island of Java asked one of the guards of the Chinese emperor's palace in the third century B.C.

"Do you have a toothache, messenger?"

"No, I don't. It is just the new emperor, who wants everyone to keep a clove in his mouth so that when we address him, our breath is sweetened."

Those venerable Chinese physicians of the Han dynasty (206 B.C. – 220 A.D.) mention in their writings the properties of the clove tree, and especially its ability to sweeten the breath. However, until the time of great journeys in the sixteenth century, the

Warning

*Those people suffering from **gastro-duodenal ulcer or gastritis** must **abstain** from consuming cloves, both as a medicinal plant and as a spice. In **high doses,** it acts as an irritant on the **digestive system,** which is shown by nausea, vomiting, and stomach ache.*

Preparation and Use

INTERNAL USE

❶ **Infusion,** with two or three cloves per cup of water, drinking a cup with each meal.

❷ **Essence.** One to three drops before each meal.

❸ **Spice.** It must be sparingly used, since a single clove is enough to spice a whole meal.

EXTERNAL USE

❹ **Mouth elixir.** Rinses with a glass of water to which some drops of clove essence have been added. It refreshes and disinfects the mouth.

❺ **Toothache.** In order to ease it, apply a **piece** of clove, or a drop of clove **essence,** on the aching tooth.

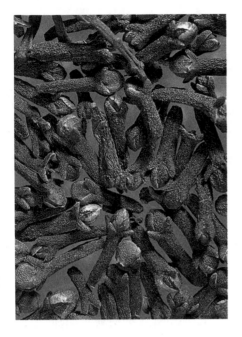

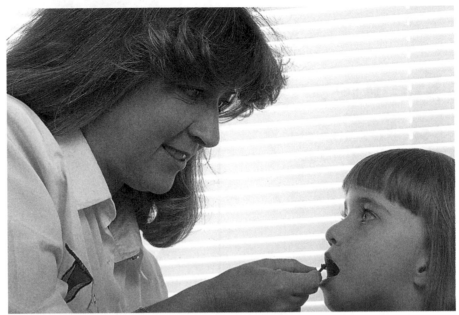

clove tree, like many other spices, came to Europe from India in very small amounts. This fact made spices more expensive and precious. Thus, one of the main reasons Christopher Columbus started his sea journey was to look for a shorter route to the spice-producing countries, and clove was one of these spices.

Tropical spices were highly appreciated in Europe. The clove was perhaps the most precious because, according to the theory of signs (see p. 48), it was regarded to be a powerful aphrodisiac. Herbalists and apothecaries of the Middle Ages and the Renaissance saw in cloves the representation of an erect penis, with the testicles at its base. Therefore, it was supposed to act on the male genitalia.

Did Columbus know this before sailing west with his caravels? He probably did. Nevertheless, the Discoverer never found the land where clove trees grew. The Portuguese seafarer Ferdinand Magellan, along with the Basque Juan Sebastian Elcano, the first to travel around the world, sailed on an expedition which in 1520 arrived at the Moluccas Islands, near China. On these islands they loaded cloves, bringing them to Spain as a precious treasure. Since then, the farming of clove trees spread to all tropical regions.

PROPERTIES AND INDICATIONS. Cloves contain 15 to 20% of essence, mainly formed by eugenol, along with small amounts of acetyleugenol, cariophilene, and metylamilcetone. This essence is what gives the clove its aroma, as well as its properties.

• **Oral antiseptic and analgesic.** The essence of clove, used as an oil, is included in *toothpastes,* orally taken *elixirs,* and *perfumes.* Its **antiseptic** power is three times superior to that of phenol. It is recommended in the case of stomatitis (inflammation of the mouth mucus membrane) or gingivitis (gum inflammation) [4]. *In local applications,* it can temporarily ease **toothaches** caused by tooth decay [5].

• General **stimulant** [1,2,3] of the body, though much milder than coffee.

• **Appetizer** [1,2,3] (which stimulates the appetite), and **carminative** (eliminates intestinal gases).

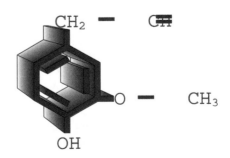

Chemical formula of eugenol, the main component of the clove essence.

Agrimonia eupatoria L.

Plants for the Throat

Sticklewort

Soothes and clears the throat

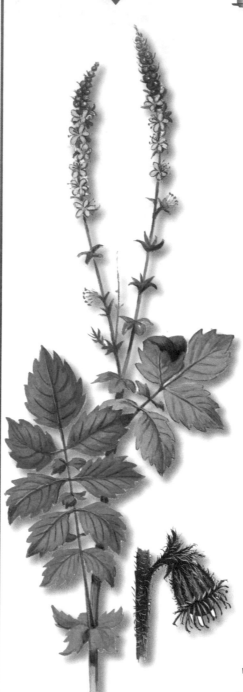

STICKLEWORT belongs to the *Rosaceae* family, which consists of more than 2000 species among which are some of the most beautiful plants. However, unlike other plants of this botanical family, the sticklewort is a plant with quite an insipid appearance, and is not exactly outstanding based on its attractiveness. Of course, as in many other matters, beauty and efficiency do not always go together.

Sticklewort has been known and used since ancient times.

Mithridates Eupator, physician and king of the Pontus (132-63 B.C.) widely used this plant, and gave it his family name: *eupatoria*.

Dioscorides and other Greek botanists and physicians applied it in compresses to war wounds. Avicenna, the famous Arabic medieval physician, also used this plant.

PROPERTIES AND INDICATIONS. The plant contains flavonoids, essential oils, and mainly tannins, to which it owes most of its medicinal effects. Tannins act on skin and mucous membrane as **astringents,** forming a layer of coagulated proteins over them, upon which micro-organisms can longer act. This fact is also the basis for skin tanning.

Preparation and Use

INTERNAL USE

❶ **Infusion or decoction** with 20-30 g of flowers and leaves per liter of water. Drink three or four cups a day, sweetened with honey if desired.

EXTERNAL USE

❷ **Mouth rinses and gargles,** with a concentrated decoction (100 g per liter), boiling until it reduces its volume to a third. Sage and linden may be added to this decoction. Sweeten with 50 g of honey.

❸ **Compresses** applied directly on the wounds, soaked in this concentrated decoction, without sugar.

Synonyms. Cockleburr, agrimony.
French. Aigremoine.
Spanish. Agrimonia.
Habitat. Common in hedges, forest borders, and slopes in warm climates. It grows all over Europe and in South America.
Description. Herbaceous plant of the Rosaceae family, growing from 40 to 60 cm high, with upright stems, and yellow flowers growing at the end of these, in racemes. The seeds of its fruits are covered with small thorns which stick to clothes and to the fur of animals.
Parts used. The leaves and the flowers.

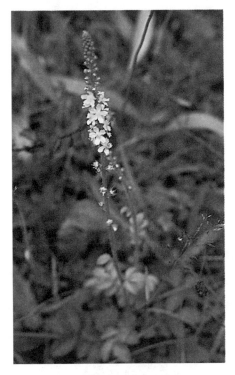

Gargles done with the liquid of a sticklewort decoction clear and soothe the throat.

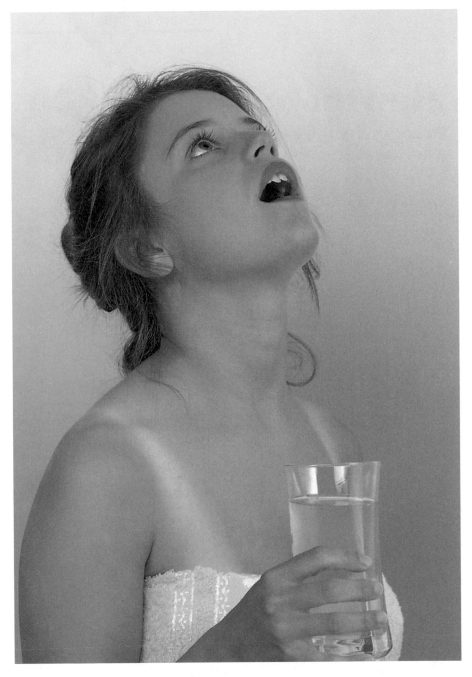

The infusion of sticklewort has an interesting **antidiarrheic** effect. It is also a **vermifuge** (expels intestinal worms) and is slightly **diuretic [❶]**.

However, the *greatest therapeutic use* of this plant is when it is *applied externally.*

Due to its astringent and anti-inflammatory effects on the mucous membrane, it is very useful in the following disorders:

• **Mouth sores [❷]**, applied in rinses.

• **Throat afflictions [❷]**: acute and chronic pharyngitis, tonsillitis, and laryngitis (aphonia). Gargles render good results in some cases, making the inflammation and irritation of the throat mucous membrane disappear in a few days.

Singers and public speakers can take great advantage of this medicinal herb, which soothes and clears the throat.

• **As a cicatrizant [❸]** in torpid wounds, sores, and varicose ulcers of the legs. It is applied by putting compresses soaked in a sticklewort decoction on the affected area. The sores then dry out, and in this way cicatrization is encouraged.

Hawthorn

Strengthens the heart and calms the nerves

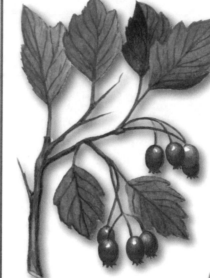

Synonyms. May bush, May tree, quickset, thorn-apple tree, whitethorn.
French. Aubépine, epinière.
Spanish. Espino blanco, espino albar.

"HOW DO YOU manage to breed such agile and strong goats?" a Greek peasant asked his neighbor, in the first century. "The Summer is already ending, and in the dry and rocky fields of the Mediterranean lands there does not seem to be much food for such mammals."

"I'll tell you the secret. Have you seen those spiky shrubs, with red berries? Try making your goats eat some, and in a few days you will notice the results."

Indeed, the neighbor's goats became stronger than ever before. They never seemed to tire, climbing the slopes under the heat of the Greek Summer. Perhaps this shepherd's ex-

Habitat. Common in all forests of Europe, and naturalized in America.

Description. Spiky shrub of the Rosaceae family, growing from two to four meters high. Deciduous, three or five-lobulated leaves; white, aromatic flowers; red berries.

Parts used. The flowers and the fruits.

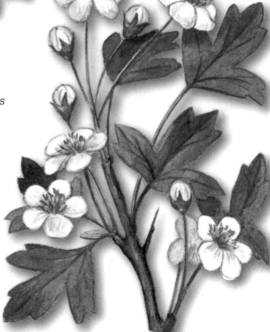

Warning

In **high doses** *(12 to 15 times more than recommended) it may produce* **bradycardia** *(slowing of the heartbeat rate) and* **respiratory depression.** *With the recommended doses there are no undesirable side effects.*

Preparation and Use

INTERNAL USE

❶ **Infusion** with 60 g of flowers (some four tablespoonfuls) per liter of water. Fresh flowers are more effective than dried ones. Drink three or four cups daily.

❷ **Fresh fruits:** Though with a low-

er concentration of active components, they are also effective, and a handful may be eaten three times a day.

❸ **Dry extract:** The recommended dose varies from 0.5 to 1 g, three times a day.

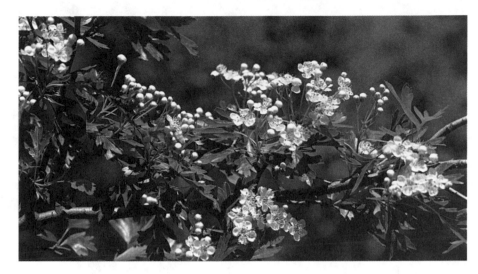

The flowers and fruits of the hawthorn are one of the most effective vegetal remedies for the treatment of tachycardia, hypertension, and other heart dysfunctions with a nervous cause.

perience was known by Dioscorides, an acute observer, brilliant botanical, and outstanding physician, who recommended this plant to give strength to the body and to heal several afflictions. Maybe its scientific name *Crataegus* arises from such an episode, since in Greek language it means "strong goats."

Hawthorn has always been highly appreciated as a remedy. However, the empirical knowledge of it, which was based upon its effects on goats, could not be scientifically proven until the nineteenth century. Jennings and other American physicians of that time studied the cardiotonic properties of the hawthorn.

At present, hawthorn is well-recognized as a medicinal herb, and is part of many *phytotherapeutical preparations.*

PROPERTIES AND INDICATIONS: Mainly its flowers, but also its fruits, contain diverse flavonic glycosides, chemically polyphenols, to which it owes its action on the heart and the circulatory system as well as triterpenic derivatives, and several biogenic amines (trimethylamine, choline, tyramine,

etc.) which enhance its cardiotonic effect. The whole plant, due to the properties of the compound of these substances, is:

• **Cardiotonic** [1,2,3]: A property attributed mainly to flavonoids, which inhibit (prevent) the action of ATPase (adenosyne-tri-phosphatase), an enzyme which catalyzes the splitting of ATP, the substance that serves as a source of energy for cells, including those of the heart muscle. When impeding the destruction of ATP, cells have more energy, thus there is an increase of the contractile strength of the heart, as well as a regulation of its beat rate. Hawthorn has the following indications:

–*Coronary insufficiency* (heart weakness), with or without dilatation of its cavities, due to myocarditis or myocardiopathy (inflammation or degeneration of the heart muscle), valve lesions or recent myocardial infarction.

–*Arrhythmia* (disorders of the heartbeat rate): extrasystole (palpitations), tachycardia, atrial fibrillation or blocking.

–*Angina pectoris:* Hawthorn increas-

es the amount of blood in the coronary arteries, and fights their spasm, which causes angina pectoris. It is a good vasodilator of coronary arteries.

The cardiotonic and antiarrhythmic effect of hawthorn is similar to that obtained with foxglove, which it can substitute with favorable results (except in acute cases). Hawthorn lacks the toxicity and the accumulative risk typical of foxglove.

• **Balancing of blood pressure** [1,2,3]: Hawthorn has a balancing effect on blood pressure, since it decreases it in hypertensive people, and increases it in hypotensive people. Its balancing action on hypertension is evident and rapid, achieving more lasting effects than with other synthetic anti-hypertensives.

• **Sedative** effect on the sympathetic nervous system (sympatheticolytic effect) [1,2,3]. It is useful in those persons suffering from nervousness that shows itself through a sensation of heart oppression, tachycardia, breathing difficulty, anxiety, or insomnia. It is *one of the most effective anxiolytic* plants (which eliminate anxiety) known.

Ginkgo

Eases circulatory disorders

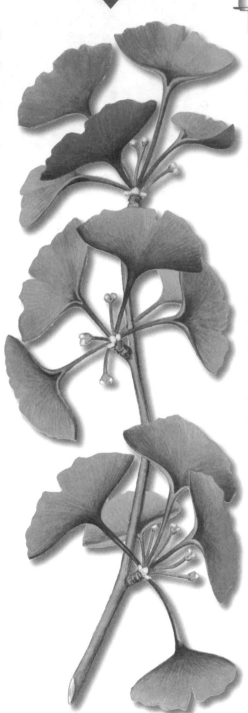

I T IS THE SIXTH of August, 1945. All around lie the burnt ruins of Hiroshima. The Japanese city has just been destroyed by the first atomic bomb. In what was formerly a park, a majestic ginkgo has burnt down into powder.

To the astonishment of the survivors, in the Spring of 1946, after the devastation, when the city is still in ruins, a bud grows from the carbonized trunk of the ginkgo. The old tree grew again, and became the beautiful tree we may see today in the center of the rebuilt Hiroshima.

The long-lasting life and endurance of this Asian tree seems to harmonize with its virtue of helping humans to confront the disorders of age.

For more than 4000 years, Chinese medicine has used ginkgo poultices to fight annoying chilblains. Its notable properties have been the focus of much scientific research, and at present it is contained in several *pharmaceutical preparations.*

PROPERTIES AND INDICATIONS. The leaves contain flavonoid glycosides, chercitine, luteoline, catechines, resins, essential oil, lipids, and some substances of the terpenic group which are inherent in ginkgo: bilobalid and gingkolids A, B, and C.

As is usual in phytotherapy, the medicinal properties of the plant are brought about by the compound ac-

---

Preparation and Use

INTERNAL USE

❶ **Infusion** with 40-60 g of leaves per liter of water. Drink up to three cups daily.

EXTERNAL USE

❷ **Compresses** with the same infusion, though slightly more concentrated (up to 100 g per liter), applied on the hands or feet with circulatory problems.

❸ **Poultices** of mashed leaves, applied on the affected area.

❹ **Hand and foot baths** with an infusion of up to 100 g of ginkgo leaves per liter of water. Apply warm or lukewarm, once or twice daily.

The best results are obtained combining oral intakes, with external applications.

Synonyms. *Maidenhair tree.*
French. *Ginkgo, noyer du Japon.*
Spanish. *Ginkgo, árbol de oro.*

Habitat. *Native to China, Japan and Korea, it is now widely used as an ornamental tree in parks and public avenues in some warm regions of Europe and America.*

Description. *Tree of the Gingkoaceae family, growing up to 30 meters high. It is dioic (with different male and female plants), with deciduous, thick, elastic leaves that when young are divided into two lobules. Its fruit is a yellow berry, which is edible when fresh, but nauseating when too ripe.*

Parts used. *The leaves.*

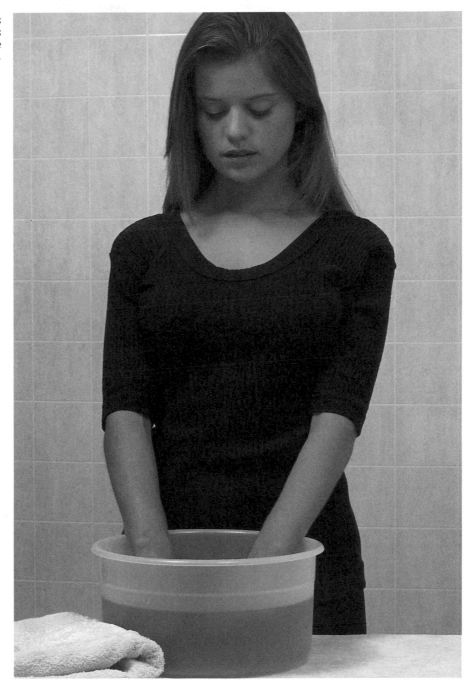

Baths with an infusion of ginkgo leaves activate blood circulation in the arms and legs. Hand baths are very effective against chilblains.

tion of all its components, and its effects cannot be attributed to any specific component.

Ginkgo acts on the entire circulatory system, improving arterial, capillary and venous blood circulation.

• **Vasodilating action.** It increases perfusion (blood flow), decreasing peripheral resistance in small arteries. It also partially counteracts the disorders of arteriosclerosis.

• **Capillary protection action.** It diminishes the permeability of blood vessels, reducing edema (accumulation of liquid in the tissues).

• **Venous stimulation.** It strengthens the walls of veins, decreasing the accumulation of blood in them, and easing blood return.

These are its indications:

• **Cerebral blood insufficiency [1]** (lack of blood flow into the brain) which manifests itself through vertigo, cephalalgia, ringing in the ears, loss of balance, memory disorders, and somnolence, among other symptoms. Those who use ginkgo say that "it clears the head."

• **Vascular brain accidents [1]** (thrombosis, embolism, etc.). It accelerates recuperation and improves the mobility of the patients.

• **Arteriopathy in the legs** (loss of blood flow in legs) **[1,2,3,4]:** Ginkgo allows patients to walk longer distances without suffering pain.

• **Angiopathy** (blood vessel disorders) and **vaso-motor disorders [1,2,3,4]:** Reynaud's syndrome, blood vessel weakness, acroparesthesia (numbness in hand and feet), chilblains.

• **Varicose veins, phlebitis, tired legs, maleolar edema** (swollen ankles) **[1,2,3,4].**

In the circulatory afflictions of arms and legs, it is recommended that the oral intake of ginkgo is combined with external applications in poultices, compresses, hand and foot baths.

Ginkgo is well-tolerated, and does not present undesirable side effects, nor does it raise blood pressure.

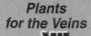

Horse Chestnut

The remedy for veins par excellence

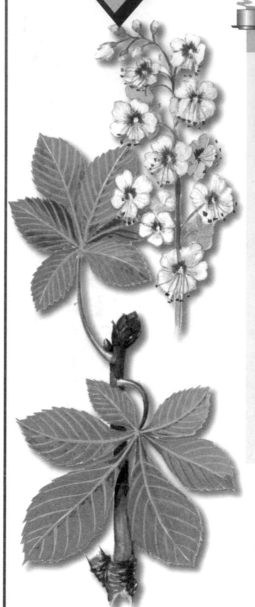

THIS BEAUTIFUL tree was brought to Austria from Constantinople, and from there taken to other Western European countries by the gardener of the emperor Maximillian in the early seventeenth century. At that time, many new plants were coming to Europe from "the Indies" (America), and this tree was thought to be just another plant, and given its similarity with chestnuts, it was called horse chestnut. Later on, it was proven to be native to Greece and Turkey.

Its name of *hippocastannum* (the Latin term for horse chestnut) brings to mind that the Turkish people gave this plant to their old horses in order to ease coughs and asthma from which old horses frequently suffer.

The fruit of this tree has a sour taste, and people should understand from it that these fruits are not edible. Poisoning has occurred, mainly in children who have eaten great amounts.

Warning

The **seeds,** that is to say, the **chestnuts,** must not be eaten since they are **toxic.** Children must be closely watched because they may mistake these fruits for true chestnuts.

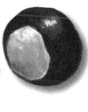
Preparation and Use

INTERNAL USE

❶ **Decoction,** with 50 g of young leaves bark and/or seeds per liter of water, drinking two or three cups a day.

❷ **Dry extract.** 250 mg, three times a day.

EXTERNAL USE

❸ **Compresses** with a bark decoction, applied on the hemorrhoids or the varicose ulceration, for 5-10 minutes, three or four times a day.

❹ **Sitz baths** with this decoction, for hemorrhoids and prostate afflictions.

❺ **Bath.** Prepare a decoction with half a kilogram of ground seeds per liter of water, boil for five minutes. Then prepare a hot bath adding this decoction to the bathtub water. This will soothe and cleanse the skin better than any other soap or synthetic soap cream.

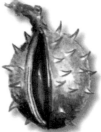

Synonyms. Buckeye, Spanish chestnut.
French. Marronnier d'Inde.
Spanish. Castaño de Indias.

Habitat. Common tree in parks and avenues in Europe and America, it is also found growing wild in mountainous forests.

Description. Deciduous tree, of the Hippocastanaceae family, with an attractive appearance and many leaves, growing up to 30 meters high, and living for as many years (up to 300) as the chestnut tree. Palm-shaped, large, toothed leaves growing in groups of five to nine. Its flowers are white, and gather in clusters. Its fruits are big, with a spiked coverage that contains one or two seeds resembling true chestnuts.

Parts used. The seeds and the bark of young branches.

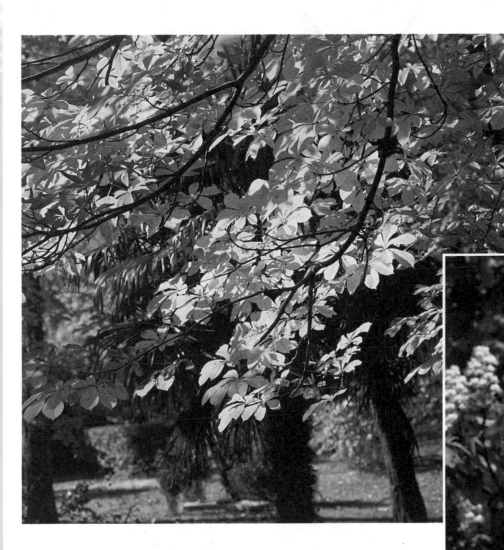

The horse chestnut is a beautiful tree, from whose bark and seeds a glycoside called sculine is extracted. This natural substance forms part of many pharmaceutical preparations due to its stimulating effects on blood circulation.

PROPERTIES AND INDICATIONS. The bark of young branches and the seeds (chestnuts) contain several active components of great medicinal value.

✓ **Aesculin.** A coumarinic glycoside which exerts a powerful action on the venous system and on blood circulation in general. Aesculin is part of *many pharmaceutical preparations,* since no synthesized substance has superseded the effects of this vegetal product. The properties of aesculin are:

– *Venotonic.* It strengthens the vein wall, and as a consequence, the veins contract and blood overflow decreases, especially in the lower extremities.

– *Capillary protection.* It strengthens the cells that form the wall of capillary vessels, decreasing their permeability, and promoting the elimination of edema.

✓ **Triterpenic saponins** (scine) with **anti-inflammatory and anti-edema** action, which are abundant, mainly in the seeds.

✓ **Catechic** tannins, with astringent and anti-inflammatory action.

This plant is very useful for all kind of venous disorders, especially in the following cases:

• **Varicose veins** in the legs, **venous insufficiency, swollen legs** [❶,❷,❸].

• **Thrombophlebitis, varicose ulceration** in the legs [❶,❷,❸].

• **Hemorrhoids.** Eases the pain and reduces their size [❶,❷,❹].

• **Prostate.** It is very effective for congestion and hypertrophy of this gland, both taken as infusion or extract, and applied in sitz baths [❶,❷,❹]. It reduces the size of inflamed prostate, and eases the expulsion of urine.

The *FLOUR* of horse chestnuts is especially rich in saponins, and it is thus used in **cosmetics** and in the soap industry [❺]. It is a true vegetal soap, soothing and protecting the skin.

Nettle

A plant that defends itself... and defends us

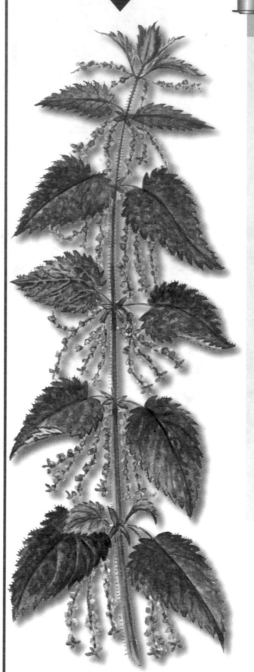

IT IS A PITY that nettles are avoided by so many people, and are even regarded as a weed. If only they knew how many virtues this allegedly aggressive plant keeps!

The nettle is one of the prima donnas of phytotherapy. Its peculiar hairs make it known, even by blind people, thus one of its common names is born: herb of the blind.

Dioscorides already praised it in the first century A.D., and his Spanish translator, Andrés de Laguna, a Spanish physician of the sixteenth century, says about nettle leaves, among other things, that "they may excite people towards lust." How could these stinging leaves be able to excite sexual appetites?

Urtications

*With a freshly gathered bunch of nettles, gently hit the skin of the joint affected by the **inflammatory or rheumatic** disorder (knee, shoulder, etc.). Then a **revulsive effect** takes place, which attracts the blood to the skin, decongesting the internal tissues.*

Preparation and Use

In order to calm those people who are afraid of this plant, it may be said that after 12 hours of being gathered, its stinging effect disappears, and the plant acquires a velvet-like touch.

INTERNAL USE

❶ **Fresh juice.** The best way to take advantage of its medicinal properties, especially of its depurative effect. It is obtained by pressing its leaves or putting it in a blender. Drink half to one glass in the morning, and another one at noon.

❷ **Infusion** with 50 g per liter of water, steeping for 15 minutes. Drink three or four cups daily.

EXTERNAL USE

❸ **Lotion,** applying the juice onto the affected skin area.

❹ **Compresses,** soaked in the juice and applied onto the affected area. Change them three or four times a day.

❺ **Nose plugging.** Soak a gauze in the nettle juice, then plug it into the nostrils.

Synonyms. Common nettle, common stinging nettle, great stinging nettle, stinging nettle.
French. Ortie.
Spanish. Ortiga mayor.

Habitat. Growing world-wide, the plant prefers humid places close to populated areas.

Description. Vivacious plant of the Urticaceae family, growing from 0.5 to 1.5 meters high. Both the stems, square-shaped, and the leaves are covered by stinging hairs. Its green-colored flowers are very small.

Parts used. The whole plant, especially its leaves.

A Good Food

The nettle is consumed raw in salads, in omelettes, in soups, or simply boiled as any other vegetable. It is a perfect substitute for spinach, even more tasty because it is less sour.

*Nettles are **a good source of proteins:** when fresh they contain from six to eight grams per 100 g, and when dried, from 30 to 35 g (a similar percentage of that of soya, one of the legumes with higher amount of proteins).*

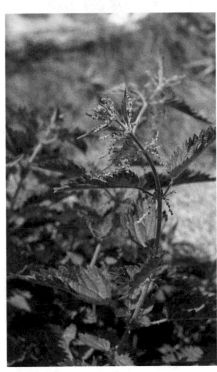

Nettles contain a high amount of iron, which, with the chlorophyll they contain, explains their antianemic action.

Messegué states that the Latin poet of the first century A.D., Caius Petronius, recommended to men who wanted to increase their virility to be whipped "with a bunch of nettles on their lower stomach and their buttocks." Urtication, or rubbing with fresh nettles, was practiced by ancient Greeks. Besides its effects on sexuality, it renders excellent results to people suffering from rheumatism and arthrosis who have guts enough to perform it.

PROPERTIES AND INDICATIONS. The hairs of the nettle contain histamine (1%) and acetylcholine (0.2-1%), both substances also produced by our body, and which take active part on the circulatory and digestive systems as transmitters of the nervous pulses of the autonomic nervous system. Some ten milligrams of these substances are enough to provoke a skin reaction.

The leaves contain plenty of chlorophyll, the green coloring of the vegetal world, whose chemical composition is very similar to that of hemoglobin, red-coloring our blood. They are rich in mineral salts, especially those of iron, phosphorus, magnesium, calcium, and silicon, which make them diuretic and depurative. They also contain vitamins A, C, and K, formic acid, tannin, and other substances that have not been already studied. The compound of these substances make the nettle **one of the plants with most medicinal applications.**

• **Depurative, diuretic, and alkalinizant.** Recommended for rheumatic afflictions, gout, arthritis, kidney stones, urinary sand, and as a rule whenever a depurative and diuretic action is required [❶,❷]. The nettle has a notable ability to **alkalinize** the blood, easing the expulsion of metabolic acid waste related to all these afflictions. The internal use of the plant can be combined with urtications on the affected joint.

• **Antianemic.** It is used in anemia caused by lack of iron or by loss of blood [❶,❷]. The iron and the chlorophyll that the nettle contains stimulate the production of red blood cells. The nettle also suits **convalescence, malnutrition, and exhaustion** cases, due to its invigorating and recovering effects.

• **Vasoconstrictor** (contracts blood vessels) and **hemostatic** (stops hemorrhage), especially recommended for uterine [❶,❷] and nasal **hemorrhage** [❺]. It is very useful for women with excessive menstruation. We have to insist that *any abnormal hemorrhage* must be checked out by a physician.

• **Digestive.** It renders good results in digestive disorders caused by atony or insufficiency of digestive organs [❶,❷]. Nettles contain small amounts of secretin, a hormone that is produced by certain glands of our intestine, and which stimulates the secretion of pancreatic juices and the motility of both the stomach and the gall bladder. This explains the fact that nettle eases the digestion and improves the assimilation of food.

• **Astringent.** It has been successfully used to calm the strong diarrhea caused by cholera [❷]. nettles are useful in all types of diarrhea, colitis, or dysentery.

• **Hypoglycemic.** Nettle leaves decrease the level of sugar in the blood, a fact which has been checked out in many patients [❶,❷]. Though it cannot substitute insulin, it allows a decrease in the antidiabetic medicine dosage.

• **Galactogene.** It increases the milk secretion of breast-feeding women [❶,❷,❹], thus being recommended while *breast-feeding*.

• **Emollient.** Due to its soothing effect, it is recommended in **chronic afflictions of the skin,** especially eczema, eruptions, and acne [❸,❹]. It is also used for **hair loss** [❸]. Nettles clean, regenerate, and makes skin more beautiful [❸,❹]. Better results are achieved if besides using it in local applications is also employed in orally [❷].

Eucalyptus

Excellent against bronchial afflictions

I N THE MID-NINETEENTH century, the eucalyptus was brought to Europe and America from Australia and Tasmania, where it grows up to 100 m high. It is one of the tallest trees known, with some examples reaching 180 m high.

The eucalyptus grows quickly, and absorbs a huge amount of water from the soil, thus being used to drain marshy lands and preventing anopheles (which transmits malaria) from reproducing.

However, this beautiful tree takes its toll on the soils where it is planted. It acidifies the soil and does not allow other plants to grow around it.

PROPERTIES AND INDICATIONS. Its *LEAVES* contain tannin, resin, fatty

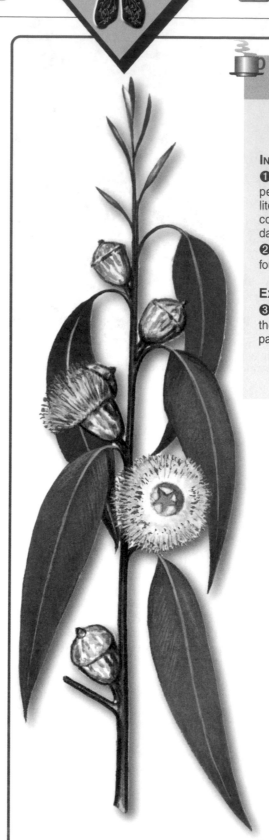

Preparation and Use

INTERNAL USE

❶ **Infusion** with two large leaves per cup of water (20-30 g per liter). Steep for ten minutes in a covered jar. Drink three cups a day, sweetened with honey.
❷ **Essence.** Administer from four to ten drops daily.

EXTERNAL USE

❸ **Vapor baths** on the chest and the head, as described on next page.

Warning

Never exceed the *doses recommended* for *internal* use (both infusion and essence), since high doses may produce gastroenteritis and hematuria (blood in the urine). However, recommended doses will not produce any side effects.

Synonyms. *Blue gum.*
French. *Eucalyptus.*
Spanish. *Eucalipto.*

Habitat. *Grown and naturalized in warm regions of Europe and America, in wet, marshy soils.*

Description. *Tall tree, growing up to 100 m high in Australia, though only to 30 m high in Europe. It belongs to the Myrtaceae family, with smooth, light colored trunk, and evergreen spear-shaped leaves.*

Parts used. *The leaves and the charcoal made from its wood.*

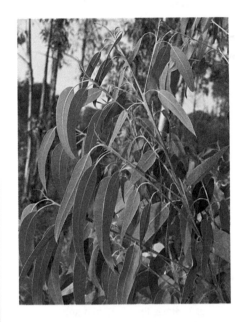

acids, and mainly essences in which its active components concentrate. This essence contains cyneol or eucalyptol, terpene hydrocarbons, pynene, and alymphatic and sesquiterpene alcohols. The **expectorant, balsamic, antiseptic, bronchidilator, and mild febrifuge and sudorific** properties of the eucalyptus are caused by this essence.

The eucalyptus is recommended in the case of all respiratory system disorders, especially in bronchial catarrh, asthma, and acute and chronic bronchitis [❶,❷,❸].

Due to its antiseptic and balsamic actions on the bronchial mucous membrane, the eucalyptus helps in regenerating damaged cells, easing the expulsion of mucus, and alleviating coughs. This is *one of the most effective plants* known for **bronchial and pulmonary afflictions.**

The *CHARCOAL* of eucalyptus is a valuable remedy for these two cases:

• Accidental **poisoning** caused by toxic substances, meals in bad condition, poisonous mushrooms, etc. It acts as a universal antidote.

• **Colitis, diarrhea, intestinal flora dysfunction, or intestinal fermentation.** It adsorbs the toxin which pathological micro-organisms produce. Its effects are fantastic.

Several Effective Applications of the Eucalyptus

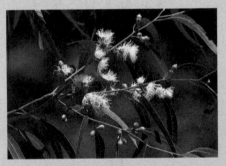

The flower of eucalyptus

Vapor Baths

*These are **the best method** to take advantage of all properties of the eucalyptus. In a bowl with boiling water, place a handful of **eucalyptus leaves,** or from four to six drops of its **essence** per liter of water. The person must sit down, with a bare torso and the head over the bowl so that the vapor reaches the chest and head. The bath should last from five to ten minutes, three or four times a day.*

This vapor, as well as the evaporated eucalyptus essence, acts in two ways.

*• Directly **on the chest skin,** favoring the elimination of toxins through the skin and alleviating lung congestion.*

*• **Inhaled** into the bronchi. To the **antiseptic, balsamic, and expectorant** properties of the essence, the **mucous effects** of the water vapor are added, then breaking down the bronchi mucus and easing its elimination.*

Charcoal

*Charcoal has many medicinal properties, especially because of its adsorption power. Both **taken** and **applied on the skin,** it has a great ability to retain toxins and germs, as well as the liquid which inflammation produces.*

Charcoal must be finely ground in order to produce the most effective action.

From five to ten g, dissolved in water, can be drunk from four to six times a day. In an emergency, one can also directly eat a piece of charcoal. It may be found in pharmacies, both charcoal powder and pills or capsules.

*Eucalyptus charcoal can be mixed with **olive oil** until a paste is formed. This is a traditional remedy to clean the digestive tract for **indigestion, diarrhea, or intestinal fermentation.***

*Charcoal has rendered surprising results in the case of **persistent halitosis** (bad breath) caused by intestinal fermentations. Take from one to three spoonfuls, 15 to 30 minutes before meals.*

Essence Against Coughs

Dissolve two spoonfuls of honey in half a glass of water, then add two or three drops of eucalyptus essence. Drink in the case of coughs caused by pharyngitis or laryngitis (throat infections), tracheitis, bronchitis, or bronchial catarrh.

Up to five cups daily can be taken, however the recommended dose for children should not exceed two or three cups a day.

German Camomile

The digestive infusion par excellence

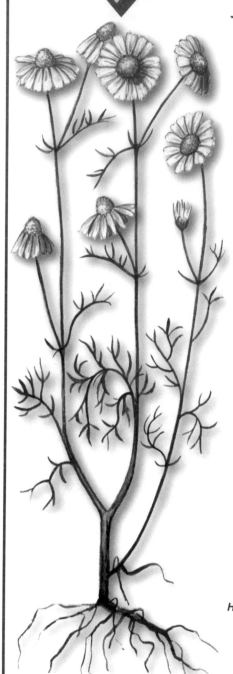

WHEN TALKING about herbal teas, many people immediately think about camomile. We could say that camomile makes *The Herbal Tea par excellence.*

"Bring a cup of camomile infusion to this patient before taking the saline solution away," the surgeon says to a nursing student.

Both of them are facing a teenage patient who has undergone surgery because of a perforated acute appendicitis. His digestive process has been stopped due to the peritonitis (inflammation of the peritoneum, the membrane covering the interior of the abdomen and its organs) produced by the appendicitis.

"Doctor, why do you always recommend a camomile infusion for post-operative patients?" the would-be nurse asks after the visit has finished.

"For many years I have been sticking to the rule of beginning oral diet for post-operative patients with a camomile infusion. My masters taught me so. Camomile stimulates the peristaltic movements of the intestine, thus recovering the digestive functions which have been stopped by peritonitis."

"How do we know that the camomile has been useful?"

"You may have observed that every day, when I pay visits to patients, I ask all of them whether they have broken wind. It may seem bizarre, however it is the best sign that the intestine is working properly again."

Preparation and Use

INTERNAL USE

❶ **Infusion** with 5-10 g of flower heads per liter of water (5-6 flower heads per cup). Drink from three to six hot cups daily.

EXTERNAL USE

❷ Eye, nose, or anal **washing,** with a slightly more concentrated infusion (up to 50 g of flower heads per liter of water). Steep for 15-20 minutes, and strain well before using.

❸ **Baths.** Add to the water of a bathtub from two to four liters of concentrated infusion. These lukewarm baths have a strong relaxing and sedative effect.

❹ **Compresses** with the aforementioned concentrated infusion, applied on the affected skin area.

❺ **Friction** with **camomile oil.** Prepare the camomile oil by heating for three hours in a double boiler 100 g of flower heads in half a liter of olive oil. Strain the mixture and keep in a bottle.

French. *Camomille allemande.*
Spanish. *Manzanilla.*

Habitat. *Common in grasslands, unfarmed soils, and roadsides all over Europe, as well as in warm regions of America.*

Description. *Herbaceous plant of the Compositae family, which grows from 20 to 50 cm high, with very branched stem, and daisy-like flowers which gather in flower heads of about two centimeters in diameter. It has a characteristic aroma, and sour flavor.*

Parts used. *The flower heads.*

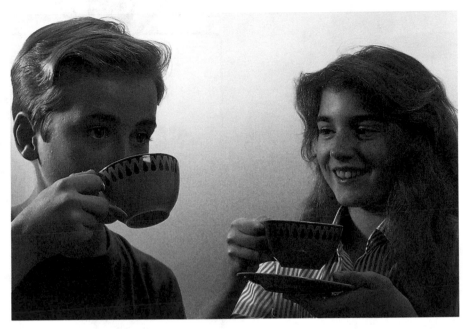

A cup of camomile after meals is a good and healthy habit both for young and old people alike.

"Oh, now I understand," the student finishes.

PROPERTIES AND INDICATIONS. The most important active component of camomile is its essence, whose main components are camazulene (with anti-inflammatory properties), and bisabolor (with sedative properties). It also contains coumaric and flavonic substances, as well as a invigorating bitter principle. The plant has many properties which have been proven by scientific research.

• **Sedative and antispasmodic.** It is useful for stomach and intestinal spasms caused by nervousness or anxiety [❶,❸]. It is also used in any type of colic, and especially in the case of liver and kidney colic, because of its relaxing and sedative properties [❶,❸].

• **Carminative and intestinal invigorating.** Although it may seem to be a paradox, camomile also stimulates the movements of the digestive tract. It is thus recommended for post-operative patients and for those who suffer from excess of gas, which camomile helps expel because of its carminative properties [❶]. Actually, the action of camomile is that of regulating and balancing the functions of the intestine.

• **Eupeptic.** An infusion of camomile is recommended for bloated or upset stomach. It alleviates the nausea and vomiting, and softly stimulates the appetite [❶]. All sour camomile species have a stronger eupeptic action.

• **Emmenagogue.** This plant stimulates menstrual functions, normalizing its amount and regularity, as well as alleviating menstrual aches. Dioscorides called it Matricaria, from the Latin word *matrix* (womb).

• **Febrifuge and sudorific.** Given that it raises the temperature and provokes perspiration, it is recommended for people with a fever, especially children [❶].

• **Analgesic.** Camomile eases headaches and some cases of neuralgia [❶].

• **Antiallergic.** Some calming properties of camomile on allergic reactions, such as asthma, and allergic rhinitis and conjunctivitis, has been proven. It is recommended for healing acute allergic crises, as well as being an ongoing treatment in order to prevent them. The best results are obtained when combining internal applications (herbal teas) [❶] with external ones (eyedrops, nose irrigations) [❷].

• **Healing agent, emollient, and antiseptic.** In *external* applications, camomile renders good results for washing any wound, sore, and skin infection [❷]. The camazulene has been proven to be effective against hemolytic streptococcus, golden staphylococcus, and *Proteus*. A camomile infusion is an adequate **eyedrop** for eye bathing in the case of conjunctivitis or eye irritation [❷]. It is also used as an anti-inflammatory, applied in compresses on eczema, rashes, and other skin afflictions [❸]. Anal cleansing with an infusion of camomile reduces the inflammation of hemorrhoids [❷].

• **Antirrheumatic.** The oil of camomile is used for massage in lumbago, stiff neck, bruises, and rheumatic aches [❺].

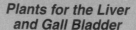
Boldo

Normalizes the function of the gall bladder

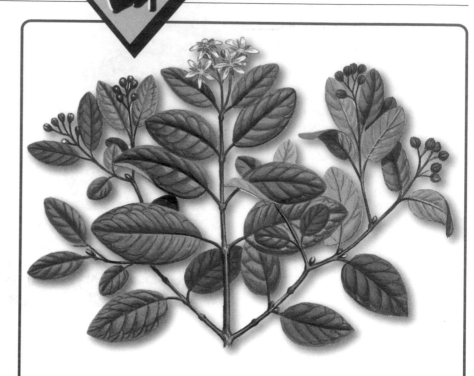

BOLDO IS ONE of the medicinal plants *most used* in preparing *medicines* for the treatment of **liver** and **gall bladder** diseases. There are several medicines, laboratory produced, in whose composition boldo is an essential part. This plant has some properties that could never be achieved by any chemically synthesized product.

It is a highly appreciated plant in Chile. Native Andean Indians used boldo because of its stomachic and digestive properties. It can be currently found in pharmacies and herb shops of Europe and America, and still with its primitive Araucanian name.

French. Boldo. **Spanish.** Boldo.

Habitat. *The plant grows wild in Chile and Andean areas of South America. It is cultivated in Italy and North Africa.*

Description. *Tree or shrub of the Monimiaceae family, growing up to 5 m high, with elliptic, rough leaves, and white or yellowish flowers. The whole plant gives an aroma similar to that of peppermint.*

Parts used. *The leaves.*

Preparation and Use

INTERNAL USE

❶ **Infusion** with 10-20 g of leaves per liter of water. Drink a cup before meals, up to four daily.

❷ **Dry extract.** One gram, three or four times a day, before meals.

Warning

Never exceed the prescribed dose *(four cups a day) since in high doses boldo has narcotic and anesthetic properties, acting on the central nervous system. These effects only occur when taken in high doses, and never with those doses recommended here.*

*Even though its effect on the fetus have not been proven, **pregnant** women should **abstain** from this plant.*

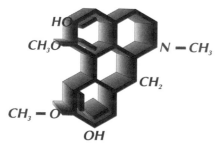

The chemical formula of boldine, the most important alkaloid of boldo.

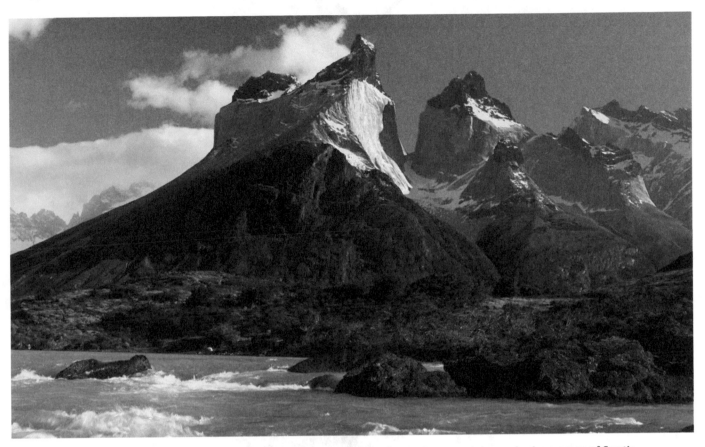

A magnificent view of the Paine Towers (Chile). Boldo is native to the mountainous Andean areas of South America, though at present it is being cultivated in Italy and North Africa. By increasing bile production, the boldo activates liver and gall bladder functions. The consumption of boldo has proven to improve skin eczemas. This is likely to occur since the plant promotes the disintoxicant function of the liver.

PROPERTIES AND INDICATIONS. The leaves of boldo contain around 20 alkaloids which are derived from aporfine, the most important of which is boldine, making 25-30% of the whole. They also contain essential oil, which gives the plant its typical smell. In this essential oil there are eucalyptol, ascaridol, and cymol. The leaves also contain several flavonoids and glycosides (boldoglycine).

The most outstanding properties of boldo are as follow:

• **Choleretic** (increases the bile production in the liver), and **cholagogue** (promotes the emptying of the gall bladder). Hence, boldo leaves are recommended for hepatic congestion and biliary dyskinesia (disorders in gall bladder functions), and biliary colic [❶,❷].

Boldo is also useful for **biliary lithiasis** (gall stones), as well as to alleviate digestive discomfort and the sensation of distension after meals, quite characteristic of this ailment [❶,❷]. Actually, boldo is not able to dissolve gall stones, or to provoke their expulsion. However, it has been proven that boldo produces changes in the chemical composition and the physical properties of the bile. Hence, it makes bile more fluid, and less lithogenic (which tends to form stones or calculi). Boldo, thus, prevents the bile from forming new stones, or those existing to grow.

• **Eupeptic** (eases digestion) **and appetizer.** Boldo is recommended for bloated stomach and slow digestion, lack of appetite, and bad breath (sour) [❶,❷].

• **Mildly laxative,** probably as a consequence of the higher flow of bile in the intestine, which this plant provokes [❶,❷].

Boldo is usually taken *in association* with other choleretic and cholagogue plants (artichoke, rosemary) or laxative (alder buckthorn, tinnevelly senna, etc.).

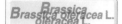   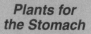
Cabbage

Heals skin and peptic ulcers

CELTS AND ROMANS cultivated cabbage, *the vegetable par excellence.* Cabbage has been used for more than two thousand years as a food as well as a medicine.

PROPERTIES AND INDICATIONS. Cabbage leaves are rich in chlorophyll, and thus in magnesium. They also contain a sulphured substance similar to that contained in mustard, as well as mineral salts, vitamins (mainly vitamins C, A, and probably U), mucilage, and an antiulceration factor still not identified. Cabbage is relatively rich in sugars or carbohydrates (7 %) and proteins (4 %), however it contains a

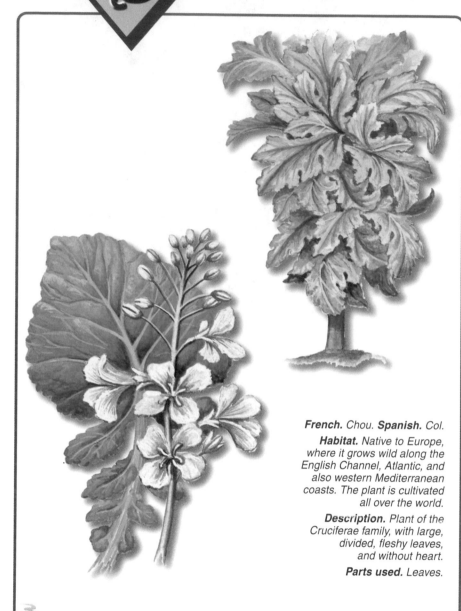

French. Chou. Spanish. Col.

Habitat. Native to Europe, where it grows wild along the English Channel, Atlantic, and also western Mediterranean coasts. The plant is cultivated all over the world.

Description. Plant of the Cruciferae family, with large, divided, fleshy leaves, and without heart.

Parts used. Leaves.

Warning

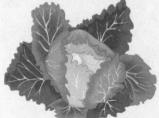

*When cabbage is **continuously consumed** for long periods, it can have **antithyroid effect,** and even produce goiter.*

Preparation and Use

INTERNAL USE

❶ Fresh plant **juice.** Drink from half a glass to one glass (100-200 ml), three or four times daily, before each meal, on an empty stomach.

EXTERNAL USE

❷ **Poultices,** prepared either with raw leaves (previously mashed with a cylindrical bottle or a rolling pin), or with cooked leaves, mixed with bran so that the mixture becomes more compact.

Cabbage leaves can be also heated with an iron, and then applied with a Band-Aid on the skin, as shown on next page.

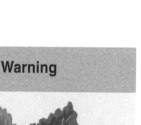

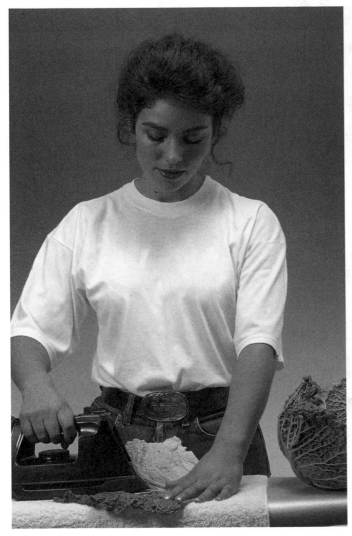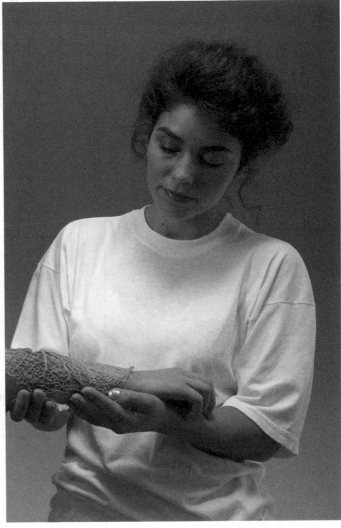

Raw cabbage leaves are heated with an iron and then applied to the skin as if they were a poultice. They have wound healing and vulnerary properties. Skin wounds and sores difficult to heal, as well as eczema and even acne, will improve noticeably with the application of cabbage leaves.

quite low amount of fats (0.4 %). It has the following properties:

• **Antiulceration.** Internally used, cabbage juice is recommended for gastro-duodenal ulcer, which cabbage is able to heal [❶]. In his work *Health Through Nutrition*, Dr. Schneider mentions experiments through which the *cicatrizing (wound healing) ability* of fresh cabbage juice has been proven on **gastro-duodenal ulcers.** After four or five days drinking a glass of juice before each meal, stomach aches disappeared. After three weeks, the ulcer was healed. This antiulcerative action is likely to be due to the still not well-known vitamin U.

• **Antianemic, antiscorbutic, and hypoglycemic** (in diabetic people, it decreases the level of sugar in the blood) [❶].

• **Diuretic, depurative,** and when taken with empty stomach, **vermifuge** [❶].

• **Cicatrizant (healing agent) and vulnerary.** Cabbage, when applied as poultices, heals infected wounds, varicose and torpid ulcers, eczema, furuncles, and acne [❷].

• **Anticancerous.** There is evidence that cabbage can act as a preventive in the formation of cancerous tumors [❶]. This is likely due to its content of carotene (vitamin A).

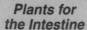
 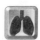
Flax

Soothes the skin and the mucosa

FOUR THOUSAND years ago, flax was already cultivated in Mediterranean countries in order to obtain textile fibers, and 2500 years ago as a medicinal herb. Hippocrates recommended it as an emollient in the fifth century B.C.

PROPERTIES AND INDICATIONS. Flax seeds contain high amounts of mucilage and pectin, which give the plant **emollient and laxative** properties, as well as mineral salts and fats with a high biological value (essential unsaturated fatty acids). Its applications and indications are the following:

• **Chronic constipation.** Flax lubricates the digestive tract, making the feces softer. Moreover, it **regenerates the intestinal flora,** regulating the putrefaction and fermentation processes [❶,❷,❸]. Its effect is thus evident, since in the case of intestinal putrefaction, feces lose their putrid odor.

• **Gastritis, duodenitis, and gastro-**

Warning

The **oil** contained in linseed flour becomes **rancid** quite easily, then produces **skin irritation.** Therefore, **recently prepared flour** is better for preparing the poultices.

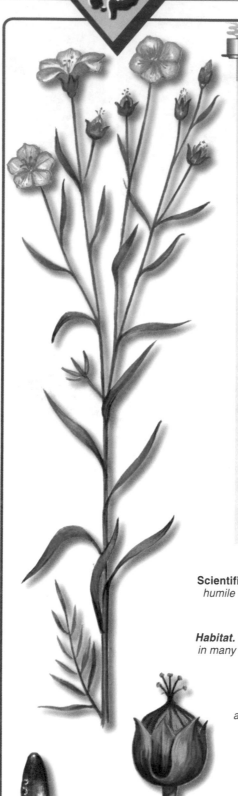

Preparation and Use

INTERNAL USE

❶ **Decoction** of 30 g of seeds per liter of water, boiling for five minutes. Drink two or three cups daily, sweetened with honey if desired.

❷ **Cold extract.** Steep for 12 hours a spoonful of seeds per glass of water. Drink two or three glasses of the liquid every day.

❸ **Seeds.** Whole seeds can be taken, chewed (a spoonful every 12 hours).

EXTERNAL USE

❹ **Poultices.** Ground linseed (linseed flour) is added to boiling water until forming a thick paste. From 30 to 40 g of linseed flour are usually required per liter of water. When applying the poultice, it is advisable to protect the skin with a cold cloth to avoid burns.

❺ **Lotions with linseed oil.** Apply directly on the affected skin area.

Scientific synonym. *Linum humile* Miller, *Linum humile* Planch., *Linum crepitans* (Boenn.) Dum.

French. *Lin.*
Spanish. *Lino.*

Habitat. *Native to the Middle East, it is cultivated in many countries of warm climate areas all over Europe and the Americas.*

Description. *Herbaceous plant of the Linaceae family, growing from 40 to 80 cm high, with an upright stem and elongated, narrow leaves. Its flowers are light blue in color, with five petals, and its fruit is a globe-like capsule with ten brown seeds.*

Parts used. *The linseed (flax seeds).*

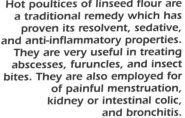

Hot poultices of linseed flour are a traditional remedy which has proven its resolvent, sedative, and anti-inflammatory properties. They are very useful in treating abscesses, furuncles, and insect bites. They are also employed for of painful menstruation, kidney or intestinal colic, and bronchitis.

Other Flax Species

All over the Mediterranean coastline of the Iberian peninsula, and in the Canary Islands grows a species called **wild flax** (*Linum angustifolium* S.), with **similar properties** to those of cultivated flax.

Cathartic flax (*Linum catharticum* L.) grows in Mediterranean countries. Its **laxative effect** is more intense.

In North America, **prairie flax** or Rocky Mountain flax (*Linum lewisii* L.) grows, another variety of flax.

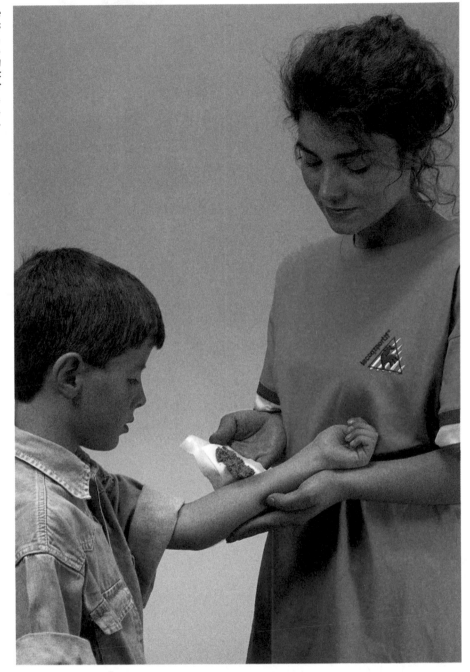

duodenal ulcer. It presents an anti-inflammatory and emollient action, which promotes the regeneration of the harmed digestive mucosa. Flax seeds should be taken in a decoction as *complement* of any specific treatment for these processes.

• **Inflammation** of the **respiratory and urinary ways:** especially bronchitis and cystitis, due to its emollient and soothing effect on the mucosa [1,2,3].

Flax *SEEDS* (linseed) can also be used as a *food.* They are especially recommended for **diabetes,** due to their low content in sugars, and its high content in proteins and fats. Linseed must be consumed by those people wanting to **gain weight** or those suffering from **malnutrition** [3].

Poultices of linseed flour are applied whenever constant heat is required: colds and bronchitis, menstrual pain, chronic aches of the abdomen (whether kidney or gall bladder aches), intestinal spasms, insect bites, abscesses, and furuncles [4].They have **resolvent, antispasmodic, sedative, and anti-inflammatory** properties, besides **retaining heat** for a long time.

Linseed oil is used as a **skin soothing product** for eczema, dried skin, mild burns, and dermatosis [5].

Bramble

Improves hemorrhoids and stops diarrhea

DIOSCORIDES recommended bramble leaves for the treatment of hemorrhoids many years ago. Its fruit, blackberries, have been used for many ages as food, being an excellent natural sweet for both children and adults.

Around one hundred varieties of brambles are known, all of them with the same properties.

PROPERTIES AND INDICATIONS. Leaves and young buds of brambles contain a high amount of tannin, which give the plant astringent and hemostatic properties. The fruit contains, besides tannin, sugars, (glucose and levulose), provitamin A, vitamin C, and organic acids (citric, lactic, succinic, oxalic, and salicylic). Their indications are as follows:

• **Hemorrhoids.** A decoction of both *LEAVES* and *YOUNG BUDS* of brambles is applied *locally* in sitz baths or com-

Bramble Buds Against Tobacco

*Smokers wanting to give up their noxious habit may try a new way to stop smoking. Put between your lips a **young bud** of bramble, and slowly suck it.*

The slightly sweet and sour flavor of these buds creates a certain aversion towards tobacco, and decreases the desire for a cigarette, at least while the bud is held in your mouth.

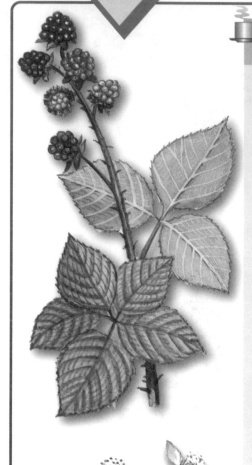

Preparation and Use

INTERNAL USE

❶ **Decoction** with 30-50 g of young buds and/or leaves per liter of water, boiling for ten minutes. Drink up to three cups daily.

❷ **Young buds** in Spring. They can be directly eaten, and provide a healing action when touching the oral mucosa.

❸ **blackberry juice.** Drink it freshly made, the dose being from one to three glasses daily.

❹ **Syrup.** Prepared by adding to the juice, two times its weight of sugar, preferably brown sugar, then heating until it is completely dissolved.

Both blackberry juice and syrup are usually mixed with the decoction in order to improve the effects and enhance the latter's flavor.

EXTERNAL USE

❺ **Decoction** slightly more concentrated (50-80 g per liter) than the internally used one. Apply it in the form of **compresses, sitz baths, rinses, and gargles.**

❻ **Poultices** made with mashed leaves. Apply them on the affected skin area.

Synonym. European blackberry.
French. Ronce noire.
Spanish. Zarza, zarzamora.

Habitat. Widely spread all over Europe, usually growing by roadsides, slopes and field borders. It has been naturalized to America.

Description. Thorny shrub of the Rosaceae family, growing up to 4 m high, with white or pink flowers, 5 petals each. The fruit consists of several small drupes, dark purple or black in color, with a seed inside each one.

Parts used. The leaves, young buds, and the fruit (blackberries).

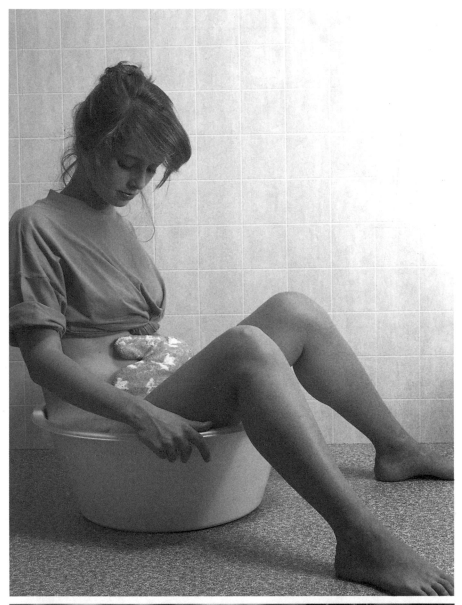

The upper picture clearly shows the right way to take a sitz bath for hemorrhoids, with a decoction made from leaves and buds of bramble.

Gentle massage with a bath glove on the lower stomach helps improve blood circulation in the pelvis, which also helps heal hemorrhoids.

The lower picture shows the delicious blackberries which are so attractive to children and adults.

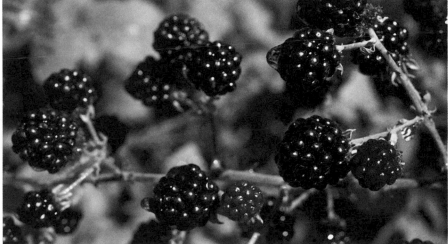

presses in order to reduce their inflammation and prevent them from bleeding [5].

• **Diarrhea, gastroenteritis, and colitis,** because of their notable astringent properties. The *YOUNG BUDS* and *LEAVES* [1] are more astringent than the *FRUIT* [3,4], however all of them are usually *consumed* together to enhance their effects and take advantage of the flavor of the fruit. **Children** suffering from diarrhea can take blackberry juice in spoonfuls [3], or the syrup made with this juice [4].

• **Febrile diseases.** The juice of the *FRUIT* (blackberries) is refreshing and invigorating, thus being recommended for weakened people or those suffering from febrile diseases [3].

• **Oral and pharyngeal afflictions.** Both a decoction of *LEAVES* and *YOUNG BUDS* [1], young green buds [2] and the *FRUITS* [3], have beneficial effects on mouth sores, as well as for gingivitis (gum inflammation), stomatitis (inflammation of the oral mucosa), pharyngitis, and tonsillitis.

• **Skin wounds, ulcers, and furuncles.** Apply compresses or baths with the decoction [5], or poultices with mashed *LEAVES* [6]. These will help with healing.

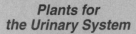

White Birch

A good remedy for kidney colic

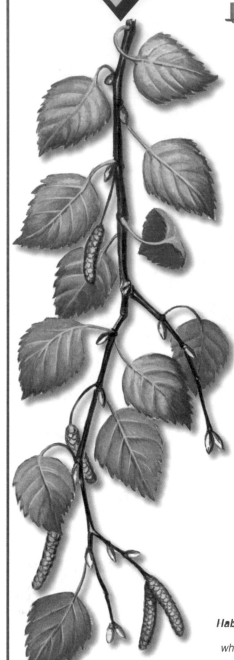

IN SPITE of the delicate appearance of this tree, its name evokes punishment applied in olden times to naughty pupils. Its fine, elastic branches have been historically used to whip rebellious youths. And still today, in northern countries, people use white birch branches to lash their legs and arms to activate blood circulation in the skin.

The great Renaissance Italian physician and botanist Mattioli christened it as "the nephritic tree of Europe."

This tree has many applications. Its wood, and especially its charcoal, is excellent. Its bark is waterproof, and with it, ancient shepherds made jars and even covers for snowshoes.

PROPERTIES AND INDICATIONS. The *LEAVES* and the *BUDS* of the white birch tree contain mainly flavonoids (miricitrine and hyperoside), which give them *notable diuretic properties* (elimination of liquids); as well as bitter components, catechic tannins, and essential oils. Their applications are as follow:

• **Edema.** They help to eliminate liquids retained in the body, especially for renal or heart insufficiency [❶].Unlike other chemical diuretic substances, white birch leaf infusions do not provoke the loss of huge amounts

Preparation and Use

INTERNAL USE

❶ **Infusion** with 20-50 g of leaves and/or buds per liter of water. Drink up to one liter daily. As its flavor is slightly sour, it can be sweetened with honey or brown sugar. When adding 1 g of **sodium bicarbonate** the effectiveness of white birch herbal teas is enhanced, since its active components are better dissolved in alkaline environments.

❷ **Decoction** of bark, with 50-80 g per liter of water. Boil until the liquid reduces to a half. Drink two or three cups daily, sweetened with honey.

❸ **Sap.** Take it after dissolved in water (in a proportion of 50 %) as a soft drink. Avoid its fermentation.

EXTERNAL USE

❹ **Compresses** on the skin, with the same infusion described for internal use.

Scientific synonyms. *Betula verrucosa* Ehrh., *Betula pendula* Roth.

Synonyms. *Silver birch, canoe birch, paper birch.*
French. *Bouleau [blanc].*
Spanish. *Abedul.*

Habitat. *It grows in the mountains of northern Spain and Europe, as well as In Canada, where it forms extensive forests, and in other cold and mountainous areas of North America.*

Description. *Fine deciduous tree of the Betulaceae family. The whiteness of its bark, which comes off in fine sheets, is the main feature of this tree. It has young hanging branches (after those it is named* Betula pendula*), with small nodes which gave birth to other of its scientific names:* Betula verrucosa*. Male and female flowers grow on the same tree.*

Parts used. *The leaves, the buds, the sap, and the bark.*

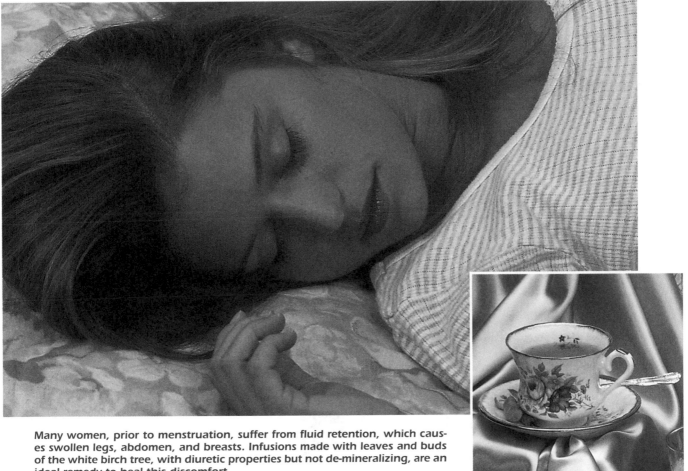

Many women, prior to menstruation, suffer from fluid retention, which causes swollen legs, abdomen, and breasts. Infusions made with leaves and buds of the white birch tree, with diuretic properties but not de-mineralizing, are an ideal remedy to heal this discomfort.

of mineral salts via urine, nor do they irritate kidney tissues. On the contrary, they are able to regenerate it and reduce its inflammation, producing a decrease of the amount of albumin eliminated through urine for nephrosis and renal insufficiency.

• They are also successfully used for **pre-menstrual syndrome [❶]**. When taking this herbal tea some days before menstruation, the volume of urine increases, and the swelling of tissues decreases, especially that of the legs, the abdomen, and breasts.

• **Kidney calculi.** Infusions made with leaves and buds of the white birch tree promote the elimination of urine sands and prevent the formation of kidney stones [❶]. It has been proven that in some cases, these herbal teas

can even dissolve calculi. The use of infusion is recommended both for nephritic colic attack (kidney colic) and, in a ongoing way, to avoid the formation of calculi.

• **Depurative.** Leaves and buds of the white birch tree have depurative properties on the toxic substances on the blood, such as uric acid. Hence, herbal teas made with them are recommended for **gout or arthritis [❶]**.

• **Skin afflictions.** Due to their depurative properties, when *internally used* they are recommended to cleanse the skin from impurities in the case of chronic eczema and cellulitis [❶].

• **Wounds and sores.** *Externally applied,* as compresses, these leaves and buds have **antiseptic and healing** properties for **wounds and sores,**

due to the amount of tannin they contain [❹].

The white birch tree *BARK*, like that of the willow tree and of the cinchona tree has **febrifuge** properties. It is taken as a decoction to decrease fever [❷].

At the beginning of Spring, before leaves grow, by cutting a branch or making a hole in its trunk, the white birch tree can provide several liters of delicious *SAP* per day. This sap has the same properties we have described when talking about leaves, as well as being a pleasant drink [❸]. Northern European villagers drink it to achieve a complexion as white and clean as the bark of the tree.

Panax ginseng C.A. Meyer

Ginseng

Not a dope... but it works!

GINSENG ROOT has been continuously used for more than 4000 years in China due to its invigorating properties.

It was introduced in Europe during the eighteenth century, and has been the issue of *many scientific studies* due to its *extraordinary virtues.*

Its scientific name of *Panax* comes from the Greek words *pan* (all) and *axos* (healing). For Chinese people, ginseng is a true panacea, able to heal a wide range of afflictions. Its aphrodisiac effects have given it a wide popularity in Western countries, in which stress, tobacco, alcohol, and other drugs have become a continuous aggression to sexual performance.

PROPERTIES AND INDICATIONS. The active components of ginseng root are so chemically complex that it has not been possible to synthesize them up to now. They are called ginsenosides, and chemically these are steroid glycosides from the group of triterpenic saponins. Therapeutic properties of ginseng are due mainly to these substances, but are also enhanced by other components: minerals and trace elements, the most outstanding being sulphur, manganese, germanium, magnesium, calcium, and zinc; vitamins B_1, B_2, B_6, biotin, and pantothenic acid; phytosterol, enzymes, and other substances as well.

Ginseng has a wide range of effects on the body [❶].

• **Invigorator.** Ginsenosides increase physical performance and endurance. This is not due to any excitant properties, such as in cocaine, coffee, tea, or other drugs, but to an improvement of metabolic processes. Ginseng

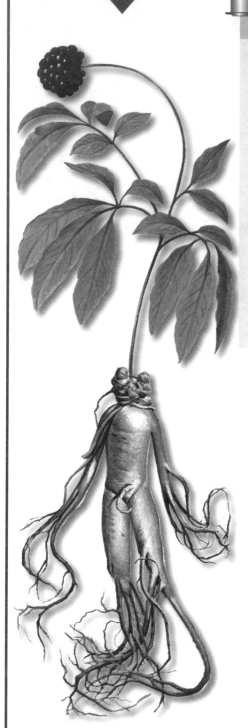

Preparation and Use

INTERNAL USE

❶ Ginseng is usually presented as **pharmaceutical preparations** (extract, capsules, liquid, etc.). The usual dose is 0.5-1.5 g of root powder per day, in a single or several intakes.

Ginseng action is slow but accumulative. Ginseng effects will be noticeable after two or three weeks of treatment.

We recommend that you take ginseng continuously for a period of time (a maximum of two or three months), and stop for one or two months before a starting a new treatment.

Scientific synonyms. *Panax schinsegn* Nees.

French. Ginseng.
Spanish. Ginseng.

Habitat. Native to mountainous and cold areas of Korea, China, and Japan, where it is widely cultivated.

Description. Plant of the Araliaaoao family, growing from 20 to 50 cm high. Its flowers grow in groups of five. It has purple flowers, which give birth to small fruits (berries). The root is fleshy, greyish or white in color, from 10 to 15 cm large, and an average of 200 g weight.

Parts used. The root after five years of age.

Types of Ginseng

There are several ginseng varieties:

- **Red or Korean ginseng** (*Panax ginseng* C. A. Meyer), which is the all-known ginseng, the richest in active components, and the one illustrated on the previous page.

- **Chinese ginseng** (*Panax repens* Max.), which is cultivated in China and Southeast Asia.

- **American ginseng** (*Panax quinquefolium* L.), native to northeastern United States and southeastern Canada. It grows wild in oak and beech tree forests.

- **Eleutherococcus** (*Eleutherococcus senticosus* Maxim.), also called Russian or Siberian ginseng, which is cultivated with medicinal goals, and has **similar properties** to those of the **Korean ginseng.**

---

speeds up the enzymatic process of glycogenesis (production of glycogen on the liver from sugar), and glycogenolysis (production of sugar from the stored glycogen); decreases the concentration of lactic acid in muscles, which causes stiffness, because of a better sugar metabolism; increases the production of ATP (adenosine-triphosphate), a substance of great energetic capabilities for cells; enhances the use of oxygen by cells; increases protein synthesis (anabolic effect); stimulates hematopoiesis (blood production) in the bone medulla, especially after bleeding. All these biochemical effects have been experimentally proven. Therefore, ginseng *invigorates but does not excite or provoke addiction,* since it increases energy production on cells.

- **Nervous system.** It has **antidepressive and anxiolytic** properties (eliminates anxiety). Ginseng promotes mental performance, increasing **concentration and memory** capabilities.

- **Endocrine system.** Ginseng has **anti-stress** properties due to its "adaptogenic" properties, because it increases adaptation capabilities of the body to physical or psychological efforts. Research conducted on animals has proven that both hypophysis and suprarenal glands are stimulated with ginseng.

- **Cardiovascular system.** Ginseng has vasorregulating properties, balancing blood pressure.

- **Reproductive system.** Ginseng promotes spermatogenesis (increases the production of spermatozoids); stimulates sexual glands (both male and female) and increases hormone production; it **increases sexual capability,** improving both frequency and quality of male erection, and promoting female genital organs excitation. It is not a true aphrodisiac substance, since its action does not consist in arousing sexual desire, but in improving function and capabilities of genitalia.

Indications for using ginseng are the following:

- **Physical exhaustion.** Asthenia (weakness), easy fatigue, lack of energy, convalescence from diseases or surgery.

- **Sports training.** Ginseng is not one of the listed doping substances forbidden in sports.

- **Stress, psychosomatic disorders.** (Gastritis, colitis, migraine, asthma, palpitations).

- **Psychological exhaustion, depression, anxiety, insomnia.** Ginseng is very useful for students during examinations.

- **Premature aging, senility.**

- **High or low blood pressure.**

- **Anemia.** Ginseng is especially useful to recover blood loss after donation or bleeding.

- **Sexuality disorders.** Impotence, female frigidity, hormonal insufficiency, male or female sterility.

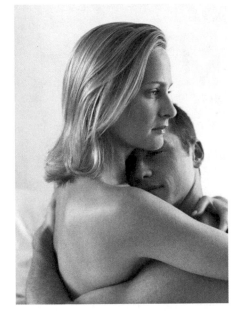

Ginseng is a general invigorator of our body, besides improving sexual capabilities.

Warning

Excessive doses can produce *nervousness.*

Do not associate it with *coffee or tea,* since it can produce nervous excitation, nor with medicines containing *iron,* because this mineral interferes chemically with the active components of ginseng, decreasing its effects.

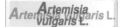

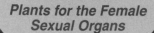

Mugwort

Regulates menstruation and increases appetite

MUGWORT WAS already used by the ancient Greeks. Dioscorides, the father of phytotherapy, talked about this plant in the first century A.D. Andrés de Laguna, a famous Spanish physician of the sixteenth century, who worked in the Netherlands, Bologna, Rome, and Venice, said of this plant that "it is called *Artemisia,* from the name of the goddess Artemis, also called Diana, since like the goddess, the plant helps women in labor, without ever failing ."

Mugwort has always been a plant used because of its effects on the female genitals. The French medical school, with its characteristic finesse, said as early as during the Renaissance that "mugwort turns women into flowers again," meaning the effects of the plant on menstruation.

Mugwort Baths

For **menstruation disorders,** it is useful to employ a combination of **oral intake** of this plant with hot water **baths** to which some handfuls of mugwort are added.

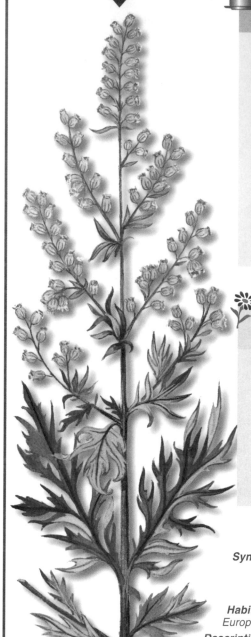

Preparation and Use

INTERNAL USE

❶ **Infusion** with 20-30 g of flower clusters or ground root per liter of water. Drink from two to four cups daily.

❷ As a **vermifuge,** that is, when dealing with intestinal parasites, the patient must drink a cup on an empty stomach, and two more before every meal, for three days. Repeat another cycle one week later.

Other Artemisia Species

In tropical areas of the Americas there are several species and varieties, very similar to common mugwort, which have the **same properties,** such as the *Artemisia dracnculuoides* Pursh., which is cultivated in North America, where it is called false tarragon.

Synonyms. *Artemisia, common mugwort, felon herb, sailor's tobacco.*
French. *Armoise.*
Spanish. *Artemisa.*

Habitat. *Very common in all kind of soils of Europe and warm climate areas of America.*

Description. *Vivacious plant of the Compositae family, similar to wormwood but taller (60-120 cm high). Its stem is reddish in color, and its leaves are silver on their undersides. Each flower chapter is formed by 10-12 small flowers, yellow or reddish in color.*

Parts used. *The leaves and the flower clusters, in summer, and the root in Fall.*

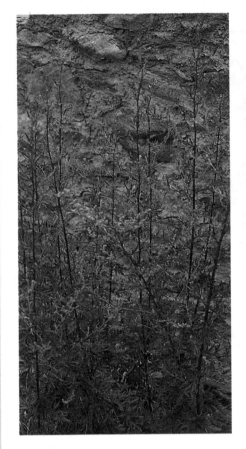

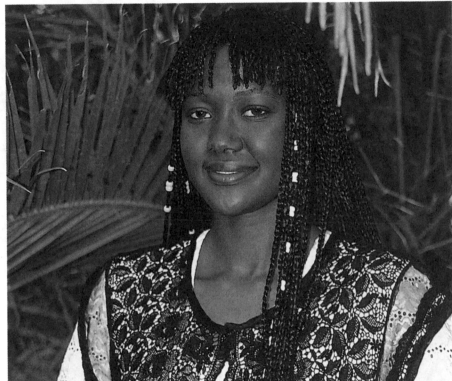

Mugwort promotes menstruation, in some cases of amenorrhea (lack of menstruation) caused by functional reasons. This plant is especially recommended for women suffering from irregular menstruation or dysmenorrhea (menstrual pain), since it helps normalize the menstrual cycle.

PROPERTIES AND INDICATIONS. The whole plant contains an essence whose main component is eucalyptol or cyneole, as well as small amounts of thujone, tannin, mucilage, and a bitter component. Its properties are as follows:

• **Emmenagogue.** It can produce menstruation in the case of **amenorrhea** (lack of menstruation) due to functional disorders. The plant also has the properties of normalizing menstrual cycle and easing menstrual pain (**dysmenorrhea**) [❶].

In ancient times it was applied as poultices on the stomach of women suffering from difficult or prolonged labor. At present, fortunately we have better remedies to accelerate labor.

• **Appetizer and cholagogue.** Because of its bitter component, it has the following properties: increases **appetite,** stimulates the emptying of the stomach (recommended for gastric ptosis) promotes **digestion,** and normalizes the function of the **gall bladder.** It also has mild **laxative** properties [❶].

• **Vermifuge.** It produces expulsion of intestinal parasites. It is especially effective against oxyuridae [❷]. In Central America, this plant is widely used because of this action.

This plant was formerly used as a sedative, to treat epilepsy and Parkinson's disease. However today it is no longer used. We have no proof of its effectiveness in these cases.

Fucus

Fights obesity
and cellulitis

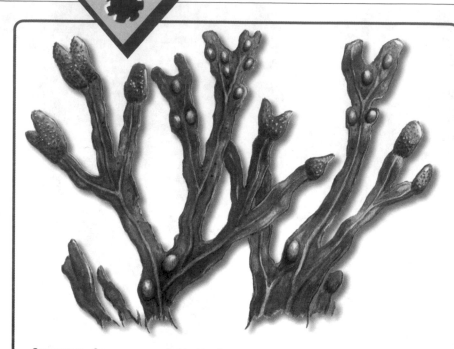

Synonyms. *Sea ware, wrack, bladder fucus.*
French. *Varech vésiculeux.* **Spanish.** *Fucus, sargazo vejigoso.*

Habitat. *Rocks and beaches on the European Atlantic coast, from Norway to the Iberian peninsula, where it is especially abundant in Galician rias.*

Description. *Algae of the Fucaceae family, brown in color, whose thallus is formed by tape-shaped sheets which stick by their base to underwater rocks. These sheets contain air bladders (aerocysts), which keep the plant upright. The reproductive system of the algae is located in its apex.*

Parts used. *The thallus (the body of the algae).*

ALGAE ARE water plants with chlorophyll or other coloring substances, whose size vary from micro-organisms (unicellular algae) to the size of an earth plant (multi-cellular algae). In China and Japan, algae have been used as food for many centuries.

Phytotherapists of past centuries, when observing the bladders of fucus, filled with air (floats), thought that, according to the theory of signs, it could be useful against diseases such as mumps and scrofula (an inflammation of neck ganglion, often caused by tuberculosis).

Modern scientific research has proven fucus usefulness in these afflictions, but the main discovery has been some interesting properties which make fucus a highly recommended algae when used against obesity and cellulitis, both ailments common among the inhabitants of the developed world.

PROPERTIES AND INDICATIONS. Fucus, or bladder fucus, when dry, contains 65% sugar, among which the alginic acid is remarkable (12-18%), as well as fucoidin (a mucilaginous polysaccharide). Fucus also contains 15% mineral salts, especially iodine, potas-

Preparation and Use

INTERNAL USE

❶ **Fresh alga.** It is taken as a vegetable, though its flavor is not enjoyable for everybody.

❷ **Decoction or infusion** of fucus dry extract, with 15-20 g per liter of water. Drink three or four cups daily.

❸ **Powder.** It is taken in the form of capsules. The usual dose is 0.5-2 g, 1-3 times a day.

In the case of **weight loss diets,** fucus must be taken in any of the listed ways, fifteen minutes **before meals.** This way, it exerts a greater

anorexigen action (which reduces appetite).

In other cases, fucus can be taken with meals, or after them.

EXTERNAL USE

❹ **Compresses** soaked in the liquid resulting of the decoction, then applied hot on the affected areas, two or three times a day, during 10-15 minutes.

❺ **Poultices** prepared with the fresh alga, previously heated in a bowl with water. Apply hot on the affected skin area during 10-15 minutes, three or four times daily.

sium, and bromine; 5% of proteins, and 1%-2% fat, as well as vitamins A, B, C, and E. Fucus is likely to contain small amounts of vitamin B_{12} since it is frequently polluted by microscopic algae which are the true producers of this vitamin. Therefore, fucus is very promising for people who want to follow a strict vegetarian diet.

Fucus has antiscurvy, nourishing, remineralizing, depurative, and mildly laxative properties, but it mainly acts as a weight loss plant, an anticellulite, and an invigorating of the thyroid. Its basic applications are the following:

• **Absorbent and anorexigen** (calms the sensation of hunger). Alginic acid and its salts (alginates), as well as the other mucilages contained in fucus, can absorb water up to six times their own weight. Because of this property, they increase in volume when in the stomach, and produce a full sensation. Therefore, fucus is a very useful remedy in treating **obesity** caused by **bulimia** (excess of appetite) [❶,❷,❸].

• **Digestive.** Fucus absorbs gastric juices, decreasing **acidity.** It is recommended to treat **gastritis and** esophagic **reflux, hiatal hernia,** and other causes of pyrosis or hyperacidity [❶,❷,❸].

• **Nourishing, remineralizing, and antiscurvy.** Bladder fucus provides mineral salts, vitamins, proteins, and other nourishing substances, which prevent, during long-lasting weight loss diets, malnutrition states or lack of these basic substances [❶,❷,❸].

• **Mild laxative.** The antiobesity properties of fucus are enhanced by its mild laxative and emollient effect due to its high content of mucilage [❶,❷,❸].

• **Thyroid invigorating.** This alga contains a *high concentration of iodine* and organic iodine salts: 150 mg per kilogram of algae (in order to obtain the same amount we would need 3,000 of seawater liters). Iodine is required by thyroid to produce tyrosine, a hormone which promotes the burning of the nourishing substances we eat, thus activating metabolism.

Because of its content in organic iodine, it is used as a *complementary treatment* of **hyperthyroidism,** whether associated or not with goiter. In these cases, *medical advice* is required. Fucus can be taken orally in any of its preparations [❶,❷,❸], and applied in compresses soaked in its decoction on the throat [❹].

• **Emollient.** *Externally applied* on the skin as compresses [❹] or poultices [❺], bladder fucus has soothing and anti-inflammatory properties, promotes the elimination of chlorine salts, and helps reduce the volume of adipose tissues. All these actions make fucus a very useful plant to treat cellulitis, wrinkles, stretch marks, and skin flaccidity [❹,❺].

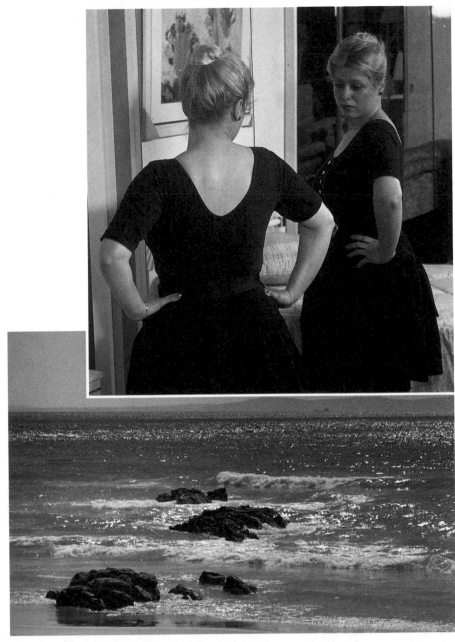

By decreasing appetite, by its laxative properties, and by accelerating the metabolism, fucus achieves an effective weight-losing action which lacks any side effect.

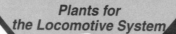
Devil's Claw

Powerful antirrheumatic

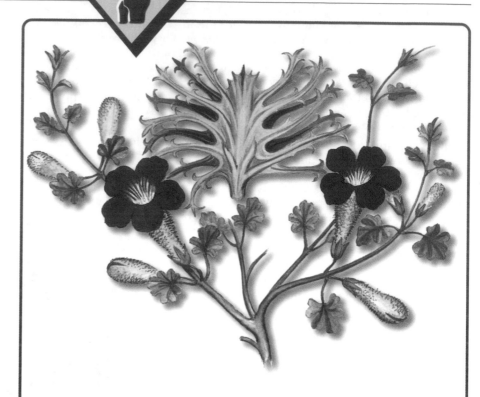

"MR. MENHERT! Do you remember that severely wounded soldier who the German physicians said they could not cure?" the native asked his master.

"Of course I remember him. Poor boy, he has died for sure!"

"But no, Mr. Menhert! He was healed with a plant the medicine men applied to him!"

"Oh, yes? I have to know which plant that is!"

The location was South Africa, near the Kalahari Desert, north of the River Orange. It was 1904, and the Hottentot uprising against German colonization had just broken out. Menhert was a German settler who worked hard on his farm, and kept good relations with natives.

"I will ask the medicine men to show me that plant which is able to heal such severe wounds," Menhert thought. "I am sure it is unknown in Europe."

However, the Hottentot medicine men did not reveal to him their secret. Therefore, the settler managed to train a dog to follow the medicine men and locate the plant. Once Menhert gathered a certain amount of the plant's roots, which was later identified as *Harpagophytum procumbens*, he

French. *Harpagophytum.*
Spanish. *Harpagofito.*

Habitat. *Native to South Africa, on the nearby areas to the Kalahari Desert, in current Namibia. It grows in argillaceous and sandy soils.*

Description. *Vivacious plant of the Pedaliaceae family, which has single* *purple flowers similar to those of foxglove. The fruit grow at soil level, and are woody, with hooks.*
The primary root is a long tuber of which secondary roots, similar to peanuts, grow. These have a very sour flavor, and are the medicinal part of the plant.

Parts used. *The secondary roots.*

Preparation and Use

INTERNAL USE

❶ **Infusion.** The usual dose is 15 g (a spoonful) of **root powder** per half a liter of water. Steep for half an hour to one hour. Drink three or four cups per day.

❷ **Capsules.** Due to its sour flavor, it is also available as capsules containing root powder. Three or four should be swallowed daily.

We recommend that you take infusions of pharmaceutical preparations of devil's claw before meals.

EXTERNAL USE

❸ **Compresses or fomentations** soaked in the infusion described for internal use, though it is better to prepare it more concentrated. Apply directly on the affected skin area, several times.

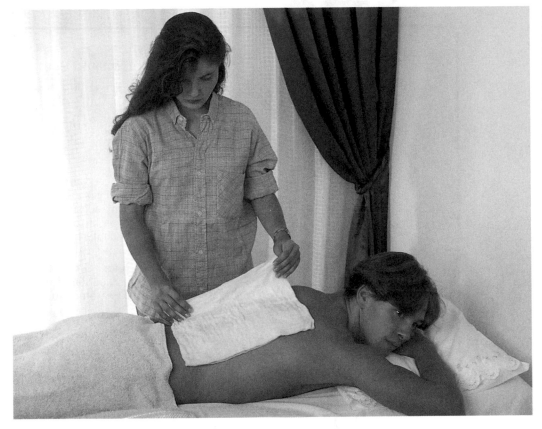

Devil's claw is a successfully proven anti-inflammatory and antirrheumatic plant which, when taken in therapeutical doses, is completely free of undesirable side effects. Therefore, it is being used more and more all the time.

sent the roots to Germany for further analysis.

Since then, the prestige of this plant has been increasing. At present it is *one of the most effective remedies* phytotherapy has in order to treat **rheumatic afflictions.**

PROPERTIES AND INDICATIONS. Since the early twentieth century, the root of the devil's claw has been deeply analyzed in depth, mainly in German laboratories, being the object of much research. More than 40 active substances have been discovered in this root, among which the most outstanding are monoterpenic glycosides of the iridoid group (glycoiridoid), harpagine, harpagide, and procumbide. The plant owes to these substances its **analgesic, anti-inflammatory, and antispasmodic** properties. Devil's claw also has **wound healing** properties, and decreases the level of **cholesterol and uric acid** in the blood. Its indications are the following:

• **Anti-inflammatory and antirrheumatic.** Devil's claw is especially recommended for rheumatic aches caused by arthrosis. Very good results are obtained for cervical, lumbar, hip, and knee arthrosis. This has been confirmed by clinic research. After two or three months of treatment, articular motility improves significatively, and pain disappears. The plant has proven useful for all kinds of articular rheumatism [❶,❷].

Unlike many anti-inflammatory medicines, devil's claw root does not produce *irritant effects* on the *digestive system*. It completely lacks any side effect when taken in therapeutic doses.

Antirrheumatic properties of devil's claw are produced both when it is taken orally [❶,❷] and when it is applied externally [❶,❷]. Best effects are achieved when simultaneaously combining internal and external applications of devil's claw [❸].

• **Depurative.** This plant promotes the elimination through urine of acid metabolic waste, like uric acid, which is the causative agent of **gout** and of many cases of **arthritis** (inflammation of the joints) [❶,❷]].

• **Antispasmodic.** It has a relaxing effect on spasms or intestinal colic, irritable bowel, and biliary and renal colic [❶,❷].

• **Hypolipemic.** Devil's claw reduces the level of **cholesterol** in the blood, and regenerates the elastic fibers which make arterial walls, being thus essential for **arteriosclerosis** [❶,❷].

• **Cicatrizant.** When *externally* applied, this plant is an excellent cicatrizant (heals wounds) for all kind of wounds and skin sores [❸].

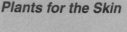

Aloe

Invigorates, soothes the skin, and heals wounds

I T WOULD BE good if you could conquer the Island of Socotora in the Indian Ocean," Aristotle said to his disciple the great King and conqueror Alexander the Great. "There, where date palms and incense grow, there is a plant called aloe which grows all over the land."

"I appreciate dates and incense, but tell me, Master Aristotle, what do you want aloe plants for?"

"Your Majesty, botanists, physicians, and wise men in this noble city of Athens have concluded that there is no better healing substance than aloe gel. The soldiers of our Army who fall wounded in the war, will find in aloe the best of remedies."

"This is very interesting, Aristotle. I want my soldiers to have the best of treatments. But tell me, how have you concluded that aloe is a good cicatrizant?"

"It has been easy, Your Majesty! We have observed that, when any of the fleshy leaves of aloe is cut, there is a quick healing on its own surface, with the aim of keeping the precious juice It contains from getting lost. Natural logic tells us that if the plant is able to regenerate the surface of its own leaves successfully, it will also heal the wounds of humans who will be treated with the plant."

At present, we know that aloe belongs to the group of xeroid plants, which close the stomas of their leaves after any cut or wound in them. Thus, they avoid loss of moisture.

Indeed aloe has been used to heal the wounds of many people throughout history. Greek soldiers, Roman

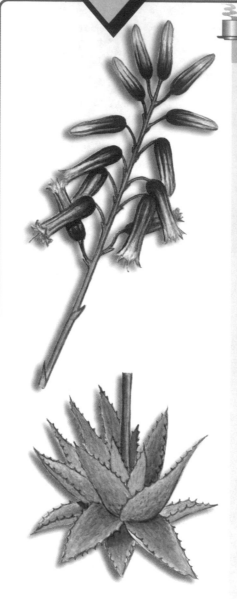

Preparation and Use

INTERNAL USE

❶ **Bitter aloes.** It is used as pills, and **pharmaceutically** made. As a laxative or purgative substance, bitter aloes act slowly, thus have to be administered at night to achieve effects the next day.

❷ **Aloe gel or juice.** Take 1-2 spoonfuls, three or four times a day, dissolved into water, fruit juice, or milk.

EXTERNAL USE

❸ **Compresses** with aloe juice. Keep them for the whole day, soaking them with juice every time they get dry. At night, olive oil or an hydrating cream can be applied, since aloe juice dries the skin.

❹ **Lotion** with aloe juice. Apply two or three times a day on the affected skin area. It is recommended that you combine its use with that of some emollient (soothing) such as olive oil.

❺ **Creams and ointments,** and other **pharmaceutical preparations** based in aloe. These usually include an emollient or hydrating substance.

Scientific synonym.
Aloe barbadensis Miller.

Synonyms. *Barbados aloe, Curacao aloe.*
French. *Aloès.*
Spanish. *Aloe.*

Habitat. *Native to southern Africa, however spread to hot and desert regions of America (Central America and the West Indies), and Asia.*

Description. *Plant of the Liliaceae family, growing up to three or four meters high, through growth of its central axis or stem. It has fleshy, lanceolated, spiked leaves, and red or yellow flowers according to its variety, which hang from a large stem.*

emperors, and warriors from many countries have been treated with this plant.

Some centuries after Alexander the Great and Aristotle, a very special soldier died on a great battlefield. Like others, he also had aloe applied to his wounded and bruised body, but after he had died. The soldier was Jesus, the Saviour and freedom fighter of mankind, an endless warrior against evil. About Jesus we can read in 1 Peter 2: 24, the following words, "By means of his wounds we have been healed." The body of Jesus was treated with aloe and myrrh, according to what is told in John, chapter 19. Three days later, he arose from death.

PROPERTIES AND INDICATIONS. From the fleshy leaves of aloe, two main products are obtained: bitter aloes, and aloe gel.

BITTER ALOES. When cutting the surface of the aloe leaves, no matter which aloe species, a viscous, yellow juice with bitter flavor flows out. It is concentrated under the sunlight or by evaporation, and becomes a shapeless mass of dark brown color and very bitter flavor, called bitter aloes.

Bitter aloes contain from 40 to 80% resin, and up to 20% aloin, an anthraquinonic glycoside which is its active component. Based on the daily dose, bitter aloes have diverse applications [❶].

• Up to 0.1 g it has **appetizer, stomachic, and cholagogue** properties, promoting digestion.

• From 0.1 g it has **laxative and emmenagogue** properties (increases menstrual flowing).

• With a dose of 0.5 g (the maximum per day) it has strong **purgative and oxytocic** properties (it provokes uterine contractions).

ALOE GEL or *JUICE.* It is obtained from the flesh of its leaves, which give an almost transparent sticky juice, with no flavor. This juice is responsible for the fame aloe gel has been acquiring for the last few years, especially because of its healing properties on the skin. This juice is formed by a complex mixture of more than 20 substances, such as polysaccharides, glycosides, enzymes, and minerals. It contains *acemanan,* an immunostimulating substance which increases defenses. Unlike bitter aloes, aloe gel does not have laxative properties.

In *local* applications, aloe can exert beneficial effects in many cases. The most important are the following:

• **Wounds,** whether clean or infected. Aloe juice is applied as compresses [❸], though the aloe flesh can be also put directly on the wound. It promotes the cleaning of the wound and accelerates its regeneration, while reducing the scar.

• **Burns.** Aloe gel or juice is applied as compresses for two days after the burn has taken place [❸]. For first degree burns, two or three days of treatment will suffice. In more severe cases, we recommend you *consult the doctor.* Aloe manages to accelerate skin regeneration in the burned area, as well as reduce scarring to a minimum.

Good results have been achieved with skin burns caused by ionizing radiations, as well as from radiodermitis (an affliction of the skin caused by nuclear radiation). It is said that during World War II, some inhabitants of Hiroshima and Nagasaki who survived the atomic bombs healed their radiation-caused burns by applying aloe flesh directly on the burned areas.

• **Skin afflictions.** Aloe juice, applied from lotion, has a favorable effect on psoriasis and skin eczema, as well as on acne, athlete's foot (fungal infection), and herpes [❹]. We recommend you take aloe orally also to enhance its effects [❷].

In children, a lotion with aloe juice is used to treat eczema caused by diapers, and to alleviate itching and promote skin healing for diseases such as measles, rubella (German measles), and chicken pox [❹,❺].

• **Skin beauty.** Aloe revitalizes skin, giving it better endurance, smoothness, and beauty. When applied to the skin, it improves the appearance of scars and cracks. It is also used for nail and hair care [❹,❺].

When *taken orally,* aloe juice has **depurative and invigorating** properties. It is used as a **digestive,** and in the treatment of gastro-duodenal **ulcer** [❷].

ACEMANAN contained in aloe juice has been scientifically proven to be able to **stimulate the defenses** of the body [❷]. Internally used, it activates the lymphocytes, a kind of cell whose main function is that of destroying cancer cells, as well as those which have been infected by the AIDS virus. Research is being conducted on using acemanan to treat both modern plagues; however without any definitive results up to now.

Warning

Aloe gel or juice can produce **allergic reactions** when applied on the skin. One out of every 200 people is allergic to aloe. If after some minutes of applying drops of aloe juice on the skin there is a slight reddening and itching, you are allergic to aloe, and will have to look for another remedy.

Bitter aloes must not be used by **pregnant women, nor during menstruation,** since it produces congestion of the pelvic organs and uterine contractions. It is advised against for those people suffering from **hemorrhoids** (it makes them bleed). It must not be given to **children. Never exceed the dose** of 0.5 grams per day.

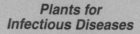

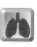
Echinacea

Heals and prevents by increasing defenses

THE NATIVES of the American states of Nebraska and Missouri used the root of echinacea to heal infected wounds and snake bites. By the late nineteenth century, Dr. Meyer, a medical researcher, discovered its properties while living among the Indians. From then onwards, echinacea has been the focus of many scientific studies, which revealed the many virtues of this plant, as well as its active mechanisms.

At present, echinacea is part of several *pharmaceutical preparations,* and it is one of the plants about which *a higher number of scientific studies* has been performed.

PROPERTIES AND INDICATIONS. The composition of the root of echinacea is highly complex. Many active substances have been identified, and could be classified according to the following guidelines:

• **Essential oil.** It consists of more than 20 components, among which the geranil-isobutirate (61 %) is important; it also contain terpenes (pinene, thujone, and others), and cys-1.8-pentadecadien, a substance which, *in vitro*, has oncolytic properties (is able to destroy tumoral cells). The essential oil seems to be responsible for the immune stimulation (increase of defenses).

• **Echinacoside.** A glycoside formed by glucose and ramnose, which has a *strong* **antibiotic** effect on several germs, especially on the golden staphylococcus.

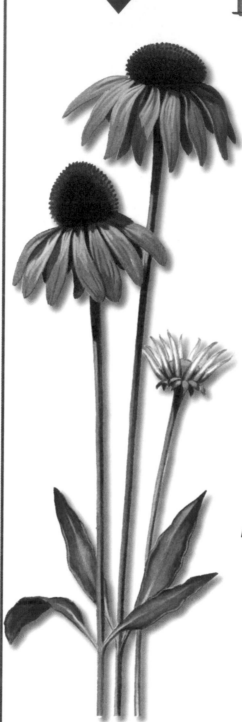

Preparation and Use

INTERNAL USE

❶ **Decoction** with 30-50 g of ground root per liter of water. Drink from three to five cups daily.

❷ **Pharmaceutical preparations.** Echinacea is usually presented in several forms: fluid extract, tincture, capsules, etc. In any case, carefully follow the instructions.

EXTERNAL USE

❸ **Compresses** with the same decoction used internally.

❹ **Lotions** with the liquid of the aforementioned decoction.

❺ **Pharmaceutical preparations:** creams, ointments, and other.

French. Rudbeckie [à feuilles étroites]. **Spanish.** Equinácea.

Habitat. Native to North America, it grows on plains and sandy river banks, mainly in the great Mississippi River Valley. It is cultivated as a medicinal plant in Central Europe.

Description. Plant of the Compositae family, whose hollow stems grow up to one meter high. It has elongated, hairy, narrow leaves, and mauve flowers which grow on the tip of the stems, and are quite exuberant.

Parts used. The root.

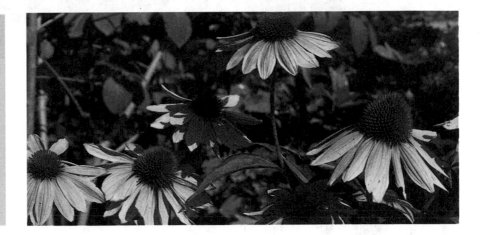

• **Polyacetylene,** which kill **bacteria and fungi.**

• An **inhibiting factor** for *hyaluronidase,* which is an enzyme produced by many bacteria. Hyaluronidase breaks hyaluronic acid (which is a basic component of the connective tissue), allowing the spread of pathogenic germs. By inhibiting this enzyme, echinacea stops the spread of germs throughout the tissues.

• **Resin, inulin, and vitamin C.**

As frequently happens in phytotherapy, the extract of the plant (of its root, in this case) is much more active than any of its active components when isolated. This is due to the interaction among its components, when some of them enhance the action of others. Also there may be some unidentified active components.

The basic properties of echinacea are the following:

• **Immunostimulant.** It increases the defense mechanisms, with a general non-specific stimulation both in the humoral activity (antibody production, activation of the complementary system) and in the cell immunity (phagocytosis: destruction of microorganisms by leukocytes). It produces an increase in the number of leukocytes in the blood.

• **Anti-inflammatory.** It prevents the progression of infections, by inhibiting the enzyme hyaluronidase, produced by many bacteria species. It also promotes the growth of granulation tissue, which is responsible for wound healing; stimulates the reproduction of fiberblasts, which are basic cells of the connective tissue and are responsible for the regeneration of tissues and scar formation.

• **Antitoxic.** It stimulates the purifying process of the liver and kidneys, through which toxic and foreign substances flowing into the blood are neutralized and eliminated.

• **Antibiotic and antiviral.** This action has been experimentally proven *in vitro* (in a test tube). However, the property of stimulating defenses is more important *in vivo* (in the body).

• **Anticancerous.** It is able to destroy malignant cells (an effect which has been only proven *in vitro* up to now).

Hence, the clinical applications of this plant are the following:

• **Infectious diseases** in general. The best antibiotic will fail when our body's defenses do not cooperate in the fight against infection. Echinacea acts on the field, that is to say, on the body suffering from the infection, rather than destroying the causative agents. This means that its action is slower, and perhaps less spectacular than that of antibiotics; however in many cases it renders best results in the middle and long term. It has preventive and healing actions, and lacks the side effects antibiotics have.

It is recommended, among other cases, for **children's infectious diseases, influenza, sinusitis, tonsillitis, and** acute and chronic **respiratory infections,** especially when these are frequent (preventive effect); for **typhoid fever;** in all **septicemia** (blood infection) for any reason (gynecological, urinary, biliary, etc.) **[❶,❷].**

It has been applied in the treatment of *AIDS,* combined with other remedies, with promising results.

• **Skin lesions.** Due to its anti-infectious, healing, and tissue regenerative properties, it is recommended for abscesses, infected wounds or burns, folliculitis, infected acne, skin ulcers, including varicose ulcers, psoriasis, dermatosis, and eczema **[❸,❹,❺].** In these cases it is applied both internally and externally **[❶,❷].**

• **Snake and insect bites.** Due to its antitoxic properties, it neutralizes (partially) the poison, and prevents it from spreading. It must also be applied internally **[❶,❷]** and externally **[❸,❹,❺].**

• **Prostate afflictions.** It reduces congestion of the prostate, and also prevents the frequent urinary infections which occur due to the incomplete emptying of the urinary bladder **[❶,❷].**

• **Malignant tumors.** Though up to now its antitumor properties have been only experimentally proven *in vitro,* there are enough reasons to think that this plant can have a beneficial action on cancerous tumors. While awaiting for new research, it must be used *only* as a *complementary treatment* of other antitumor treatments **[❶,❷].**

Books on Health

Encyclopedia of Medicinal Plants
2 Volumes

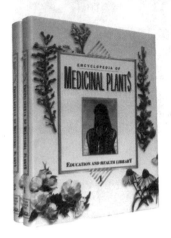

This is a complete, up-to-date, and scientific encyclopedia, based on rigorous botanical, pharmaceutical, and chemical research. More than 470 plants botanically described and classified by diseases. Numerous natural treatments are explained with clear illustrations and simple language. Numerous charts that describe the most frequent disorders and the plants that possess the active principles to correct them. 795 pages in two volumes, hardcover.

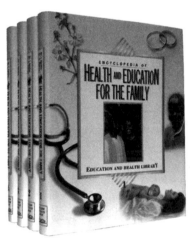

Encyclopedia of Health and Education
for the Family
4 Volumes

A medical-educational encyclopedia for the whole family, these books cover more than 400 diseases with their natural, pharmacological, and/or surgical treatments. The Encyclopedia contains numerous tips on educational topics for the whole family. Offering practical orientation from medics, psychologists, and educators to help you maintain and improve your physical, mental, and social health. 1,539 pages in four volumes, hardcover.

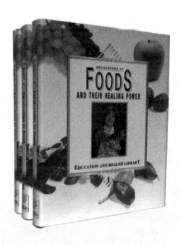

Encyclopedia of Foods and their Healing Power
3 Volumes

This is a modern and concise encyclopedia that presents the latest research on food science, nutrition, and dietetics. With almost 700 foods from 5 continents described and around 300 recipes, the information contained in this encyclopedia is based on the latest research at the main universities and research centers of Europe, America, and other continents. 1,278 pages in three volumes, hardcover.

For more information, write: Home Health Education Service, PO Box 1119, Hagerstown, MD, 21741-1119

MORE *F*AMILY READING

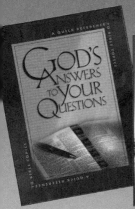

**God's Answers
to Your Questions**
You ask the
questions; it points
you to Bible texts
with the answers

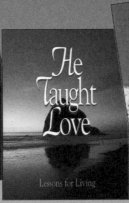

**He Taught
Love**
The true meaning
hidden within the
parables of Jesus

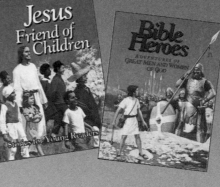

**Jesus, Friend
of Children**
Favorite
chapters from
The Bible Story

Bible Heroes
A selection
of the most
exciting adven-
tures from
The Bible Story

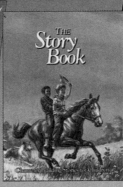

The Storybook
Excerpts from
Uncle Arthur's
Bedtime Stories

My Friend Jesus
Stories for
preschoolers from
the life of Christ,
with activity pages

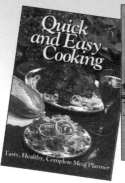

**Quick and Easy
Cooking**
Plans for complete,
healthful meals

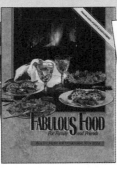

**Fabulous Food for
Family and
Friends**
Complete menus
perfect for
entertaining

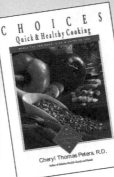

**Choices:
Quick and
Healthy
Cooking**
Healthy meal
plans you can
make in a hurry

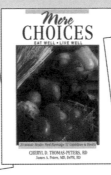

**More Choices
for a Healthy,
Low-Fat You**
All-natural meals
you can make in
30 minutes

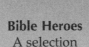

**Tasty Vegan
Delights**
Exceptional
recipes without
animal fats or
dairy products

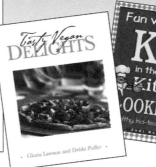 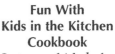

**Fun With
Kids in the Kitchen
Cookbook**
Let your kids help
with these healthy
recipes

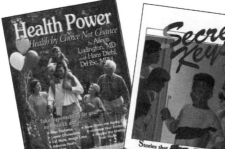 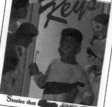 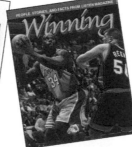

Health Power
Choices you can make
that will revolutionize
your health

Secret Keys
Character-building
stories for
children

Winning
Gives teens
good reasons to
be drug-free

FOR MORE INFORMATION:
- mail the attached card
- or write
  Home Health Education Service
  P.O. Box 1119
  Hagerstown, MD 21741
- or visit **www.thebiblestory.com**